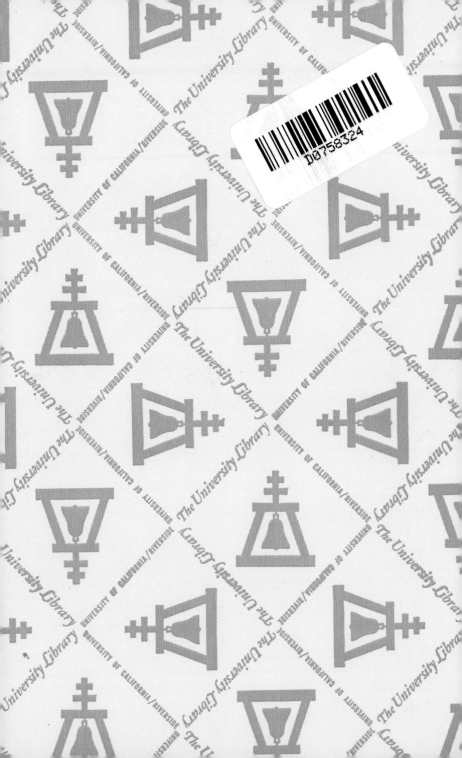

# Cancer pain relief and palliative care in children

World Health Organization
Geneva
1998

WHO Library Cataloguing in Publication Data

Cancer pain relief and palliative care in children.

  Companion volume to: Cancer pain relief, with a guide to opioid availability.

  1. Neoplasms – in infancy and childhood    2. Neoplasms – therapy
  3. Pain – in infancy and childhood    4. Pain – therapy
  5. Palliative care – in infancy and childhood    6. Narcotherapy –
  in infancy and childhood

ISBN 92 4 154512 7              (NLM Classification: QZ 275)

Typeset in Switzerland
Printed in England
97/11427 – Strategic/Clays – 12000

# Contents

# Preface

In 1993, WHO and the International Association for the Study of Pain (IASP) invited experts in the fields of oncology, anaesthesiology, neurology, paediatrics, nursing, palliative care, psychiatry, psychology, and pastoral care to attend a conference on the management of paediatric cancer pain and palliative care. At this meeting, in Gargonza, Italy, it was agreed that pain relief should be regarded as an essential component of cancer care and that, with commitment and the appropriate use of available technology, most children with cancer throughout the world can receive both pain relief and palliative care — even if cure is impossible.

A number of fears and misunderstandings have led to inadequate pain control in children with cancer. These include:

- fear of drug "addiction", in the lay sense of the term, which has led to the limited administration of opioid analgesics, generally as a last resort, with the result that children have been deprived of the potent drugs that can effectively relieve severe cancer pain;

- misunderstanding of the pharmacodynamics and pharmacokinetics of opioid analgesics in children and consequent use of inadequate doses, at inappropriate intervals, by unnecessarily painful or less effective routes;

- lack of knowledge about the nature of children's perception of pain and illness, so that some individuals responsible for treating children with cancer fail to evaluate all the factors that cause or contribute to pain and thus fail to treat it adequately;

- lack of information about the simple behavioural, cognitive, and supportive techniques that can reduce pain, so that health professionals cannot teach these valuable techniques to children or their families.

It is for reasons such as these that it was considered necessary to produce a book dealing exclusively with cancer pain relief and palliative care in children. The intention is to clear up the misunderstandings and provide the missing information, and thus offer a comprehensive guide to pain management in childhood cancer.

The guidelines contained in this book have been approved by both WHO and IASP. Although intended largely for health-care workers with primary responsibility for treating children with cancer, the book should find wider readership among policy-makers and those concerned with the legislation that governs availability of opioid analgesics. It is a companion volume to WHO's *Cancer pain relief*, published in its second edition in 1996 and containing a guide to opioid availability. As noted in that publication, management of cancer pain should not be undertaken in isolation, but as part of comprehensive palliative care. Relief of other cancer symptoms, and of psychological, social, and spiritual problems, is paramount. Attempting to relieve pain without addressing the patient's non-physical concerns is likely to lead to frustration and failure.

# Acknowledgements

The financial support and the assistance of the Livia Benini Foundation of Florence, Italy, in arranging the meeting that was the basis for this book are acknowledged with gratitude.

Financial support for the meeting was also kindly provided by the following organizations:

American Italian Foundation, New York, NY, USA

Canadian Cancer Society, Toronto, Canada

Cancer Relief India, London, England

Gimbel Foundation, New York, NY, USA

Health and Welfare Canada, Ottawa, Canada

Knoll Pharmaceutical Company, Toronto, Canada

Kornfeld Foundation, New York, NY, USA

Laboratoire UPSA, Paris, France

Richwood Pharmaceutical Company, Cincinnati, OH, USA

U.S. Cancer Pain Relief Committee, Madison, WI, USA

WHO Collaborating Centre on Cancer Control and Palliative Care, Milan, Italy

WHO Collaborating Centre for Cancer Pain Relief and Quality of Life, Saitama, Japan

WHO Collaborating Centre for Cancer Pain Research and Education, New York, NY, USA

The World Health Organization gratefully acknowledges the generous financial contribution made by the Open Society Institute of New York towards the publication of the book.

The following individuals attended the meeting in Gargonza, Italy, and their valuable contributions are acknowledged with thanks:

Dr F. Benini, Department of Paediatrics, University of Padua, Padua, Italy.

Dr G. Benini, Department of Paediatrics, University of Florence, Florence, Italy.

Dr C.B. Berde, Pain Treatment Service, Children's Hospital, Boston, MA, USA.

Ms M. Callaway, WHO Collaborating Centre for Cancer Pain Research and Education, Memorial Sloan-Kettering Cancer Center, New York, NY, USA.

Dr J. Eland, College of Nursing, University of Iowa, Iowa City, IA, USA.

Dr K.M. Foley, WHO Collaborating Centre for Cancer Pain Research and Education, Memorial Sloan-Kettering Cancer Center, New York, NY, USA.

Dr S. Fowler-Kerry, College of Nursing, University of Saskatchewan, Saskatoon, Canada.

Dr G. Frager, IWK Grace Health Centre, Halifax, Nova Scotia, Canada.

Dr Y. Kaneko, Pediatric Service, Hematology Clinic, Saitama Cancer Center, Saitama, Japan.

Dr P.A. Kurkure, Department of Medical Oncology, Tata Memorial Hospital, Bombay, India.

Dr L. Kuttner, Clinical Psychologist, Vancouver, BC, Canada.

Dr I. Martinson, School of Nursing, University of California, San Francisco, CA, USA.

Rev. Dr T. McDonnell, Maryknoll Fathers and Brothers, Nairobi, Kenya.

Dr P.A. McGrath, Pediatric Pain Program, Child Health Research Institute, University of Western Ontario, London, Ontario, Canada.

Dr P.J. McGrath, Clinical Psychology, Dalhousie University, Halifax, Nova Scotia, Canada.

Ms L.A.N. Nesbitt, Thomas Barnardo House, Nairobi, Kenya.

Dr E.M. Pichard-Léandri, Pain Treatment Unit, Gustave-Roussy Institute, Villejuif, France.

Dr L. Saita, Pain Therapy and Palliative Care Division, National Cancer Institute, Milan, Italy.

Dr N.L. Schechter, University of Connecticut, School of Medicine/ St Francis Hospital, Hartford, CT, USA.

Dr B.S. Shapiro, Pain Management Service, Children's Hospital of Philadelphia, Philadelphia, PA, USA.

Dr J. Stjernswärd, Cancer, World Health Organization, Geneva, Switzerland.

Ms N. Teoh, Cancer, World Health Organization, Geneva, Switzerland.

Dr V. Ventafridda, WHO Collaborating Centre on Cancer Control and Palliative Care, European Institute of Oncology, Milan, Italy.

Thanks are also due to Dr A.M. Sbanotto of the European Institute of Oncology, Milan, Italy and to Drs Berde, Frager, and Schechter for their help in preparation and review of the text.

Dr K. Sikora, Chief, WHO Programme on Cancer Control, Lyon, France, coordinated the final revision of the text.

# Introduction

Children with cancer do not need to suffer unrelieved pain. Existing knowledge provides a basic approach for relieving cancer pain that can be implemented in developed and developing countries alike. Effective pain management and palliative care are major priorities of the WHO cancer programme, together with primary prevention, early detection, and treatment of curable cancers.

Pain management must begin when a child is first diagnosed with cancer and must continue throughout the course of the illness. Analgesic and anaesthetic drug therapies are essential in controlling pain and should be combined with appropriate psychosocial, physical, and supportive approaches to this problem.

## Extent of the problem

Cancer is a major world health problem with wide geographical variations in its incidence. Out of every one million children aged 0–14 years, approximately 130 develop cancer every year ( 1 ). In developed countries cancer is the leading cause of death from disease in 1–14-year-olds ( 1 ). Approximately 67% of children can be cured if the disease is diagnosed early and appropriately treated ( 2 ), although the cure rate depends upon the specific type of cancer. Unfortunately, however, most children with cancer do not receive curative therapies because they live in developing countries ( 3 ): the disease is usually advanced by the time of diagnosis and curative therapies are frequently unavailable. Palliation of pain and other symptoms is a component of care for all children with cancer. For some children, the emphasis of care may be primarily one of palliation.

During the course of their illness, almost all children with cancer experience some pain, caused either directly by the disease or by invasive procedures, treatments, or psychological distress. At present, there are no accurate figures on the worldwide magnitude of different types of cancer pain in children because countries differ widely in their diagnostic capabilities and reporting systems. However, recent documentation of childhood cancer pain within specific treatment centres in developed countries indicates that all children with cancer do experience pain related to their disease and/or treatment, with more than 70% of them suffering from severe pain at some point (4). Although the means exist for its effective relief, children's pain is often not recognized or, if recognized, may be inadequately treated, even when sufficient resources are available.

Unrelieved pain places an enormous burden on children and families. Children become afraid of future pain, and develop mistrust and fear of hospitals, medical staff, and treatment procedures. They become irritable, anxious, and restless in response to pain and may also experience night terrors, flashbacks, sleep disturbance, and eating problems. Children with uncontrolled pain may feel victimized, depressed, isolated, and lonely, and their capacity to cope with cancer treatment may be impaired.

Parents and other close relatives of a child in pain often feel angry and distrustful towards the medical system, and experience depression and guilt about being unable to prevent the pain. They may even come into conflict with the child and will have disturbing memories of his or her pain and suffering.

Poorly managed pain affects health care workers: it numbs their compassion, creates guilt, and encourages denial that children are suffering. Its effects on children and their families are enduring, and children can suffer from post-traumatic stress symptoms, phobic reactions, depression, and pain years after the end of treatment.

## The nature of children's pain

Children understand the basic concept of pain at a very young age and can describe both its emotional and physical aspects. Nonetheless, pain is a difficult sensation to define simply and precisely; the definition provided by IASP is *"an unpleasant sensory and emotional experience associated with actual or potential tissue damage, or described in terms of such damage"* (5).

Pain is always subjective; each individual learns the application of the word through experiences related to injury in early life. Physical pain is unquestionably a sensation in a part, or parts, of the body, but it is always unpleasant and is therefore also an emotional experience. New information about the nature of pain has led to an improved understanding of how children experience it and how their suffering can be alleviated. The pain system is now known to be much more variable and complex than was previously believed.

Simply expressed, tissue damage causes activity in specialized receptors and nerves that can lead to pain, but this nerve activity can be modified before the information is relayed to the brain. Activity in peripheral non-pain nerves (e.g. those stimulated by touch) can inhibit the effects of pain nerve activity at a spinal level. Also, activity in central nerves descending from the brain (i.e. nerve systems that are activated by thoughts, behaviours, and emotions) can inhibit the activity caused by tissue damage at spinal levels. Thus, the spinal cord provides a complex "gating" system for enhancing or blocking pain signals (6).

Pain in children with cancer is usually related to the disease or to its treatment. It depends not only upon the specific source of physical damage, but also upon the complex interactions among peripheral pain and non-pain nerves, and upon activity in central descending pain-inhibitory systems. Thus, the same type of tissue damage can cause pain of different nature or severity in different children or in the same child at different times.

In addition, environmental, developmental, behavioural, psychological, familial, and cultural factors profoundly affect pain and suffering (7–11). The physical environment and the attitudes and behaviour of caregivers, as well as children's own behaviour, thoughts, and emotional states, can profoundly increase or decrease children's cancer pain.

# PART I

# Comprehensive care for children with cancer

# Introduction

Comprehensive care of children with cancer includes curative therapies, pain management, and symptom control, plus compassionate support both for the children and for their families. The diagnosis of cancer abruptly changes the lives of all family members. The initial reactions of parents are disbelief, anguish, and despair, and the sudden feeling that they have little control over their lives or the life of their child. They become anxious, frightened, and uncertain about the future; normal life temporarily stops. Parents and children therefore require special psychosocial and spiritual support to help them learn to live with cancer. In some specialized cancer centres, this type of support is provided from the time of diagnosis throughout the child's medical care. Other centres, however, continue to focus exclusively on the medical management of the disease and show little understanding of the importance of adequate analgesia and psychosocial and spiritual support. As a result, many children with cancer may not receive comprehensive care even though this should be possible in almost all countries.

It is essential for health providers to recognize that children, their parents, and their siblings will all react to a potentially fatal illness differently, according to their own personalities, past experiences, and perception of the disease. To support and assist children effectively, it is important to know them and their families, their beliefs about life and death, and their current sources of emotional support. Such an approach is central to the concept of palliative care.

# Palliative care

In a medical context, the verb "to palliate" means to mitigate, to alleviate, to lessen the severity of (pain or disease), or to give temporary relief. When palliative medicine was recognized as a medical speciality in 1987, it was defined as *"the study and management of patients with active, progressive, far-advanced disease for whom the prognosis is limited and the focus of care is the quality of life"* ( *12*). The care that can be offered by a team of health professionals, members of the religious community, and volunteers to children with cancer is perhaps better summarized by WHO ( *13*) as that in which:

> *... control of pain, of other symptoms, and of psychological, social and spiritual problems, is paramount. The goal of palliative care is achievement of the best quality of life for patients and their families. Many aspects of palliative care are also applicable earlier in the course of the illness in conjunction with anticancer treatment.*

Palliative care is the active total care of the child's body, mind and spirit, and also involves giving support to the family. It begins when cancer is diagnosed, and continues regardless of whether or not a child receives treatment directed at the disease. Health providers must evaluate and alleviate a child's physical, psychological, and social distress. Effective palliative care requires a broad multidisciplinary approach that includes the family and makes use of available community resources ( *14*); it can be successfully implemented even if resources are limited. It can be provided in tertiary care facilities, in community health centres and even in children's homes.

Nothing would have a greater impact on the quality of life of children with cancer than the dissemination and implementation of the current principles of palliative care, including pain relief and symptom control.

8

# Types of cancer pain in children

Almost all children with cancer experience pain at some point during their illness — pain caused by the cancer itself, by treatments, and by invasive diagnostic or therapeutic procedures, as well as incidental pain from unrelated causes (see Table 1) (*15, 16*). Malignancies in childhood differ from those in adults in that haematological neoplasms are more common than solid tumours. When curative therapies are available, such neoplasms often respond rapidly to treatment and

Table I
**Major types of pain in childhood cancer**

*Caused by disease:*
Tumour involvement of bone
Tumour involvement of soft tissue
Tumour involvement of viscera
Tumour involvement of central or peripheral nervous system, including pain
    from spinal cord compression

*Caused by anticancer treatment*
Postoperative pain
Radiation-induced dermatitis
Gastritis from repeated vomiting
Prolonged post-lumbar puncture headache
Corticosteroid-induced bone changes
Neuropathy, including phantom limb pain and drug-induced neuropathy
Infection
Mucosal damage
Mucositis

*Caused by procedures*
Finger prick
Venepuncture
Injection
Lumbar puncture
Bone marrow aspiration and biopsy

*Incidental*
Trauma
Usual childhood pains

children frequently experience prompt pain relief, although some may suffer persistent pain for a lengthy period. When curative therapies are not available, death is often rapid.

Disease-related pain can be acute or chronic and is usually caused by direct invasion of anatomical structures, by pressure on (or entrapment of) nerves, or by obstruction. The most common childhood malignancies, such as leukaemia, lymphoma, and neuroblastoma, often produce diffuse bone and joint pain. Leukaemia and lymphomatous disease, together with brain tumours and certain solid tumours, can produce headaches resulting from meningeal irritation and obstruction with increased intracranial pressure.

Treatment-related pain can be either a direct result of physical interventions or a side-effect of treatment. For many children, these pains are the worst part of their disease, accounting for most of the pain they experience and intensifying as repeated procedures are required (16, 17). Physical interventions for diagnostic or therapeutic purposes include procedures such as bone-marrow aspirations, lumbar punctures, or venepunctures, and surgical operations such as amputations. Children can also experience a great deal of pain caused by the side-effects of chemotherapy, radiation therapy, and medications, including mucositis, neuropathies, radiation reactions, and infections resulting from neutropenia.

---

In the developed world, the major sources of pain in children's cancer are diagnostic and therapeutic procedures. In the developing world, most pain is disease-related.

---

Children can also experience pain after the disease has been controlled; this is caused by the late effects of cancer and its treatment. Pains of this type may become more common as the childhood cancer survival rate continues to rise with improved treatment.

# PART 2
# Therapeutic strategies

# Introduction

Because of its complexity, children's cancer pain must be treated within a broad context, and the expertise of different disciplines is often beneficial. Ideally, the health-care setting should be sensitive to the developmental needs of children, the staff skilled in working with children, and parents actively involved in their children's care. Unlike adults, children cannot independently seek pain relief and are therefore vulnerable; they need adults to recognize their pain before they can receive appropriate treatment.

Comprehensive management of cancer in children includes active treatment of the disease as well as pharmacological and non-pharmacological interventions to reduce pain and suffering. These approaches can be incorporated into a flexible programme for children in which parents, siblings, and other significant family and community members assist the health-care team.

The proposed therapeutic strategy for managing cancer pain in children is shown in Fig. 1. Management of such pain begins with a thorough physical examination and assessment of the sensory characteristics of the pain (location, quality, intensity, duration), its primary underlying etiology, and the secondary contributing physical and psychological factors. For effective pain relief, treatments must be targeted to both the primary pain source and the various secondary sources. The chronology of the disease, previous therapy, and the child's individual characteristics must be considered carefully, to allow the selection of the most appropriate drug and non-drug therapies. While complete relief of pain may not always be possible, the strategy shown in Fig. 1 — following the basic principles of pain management — will significantly improve pain control for all children.

Fig. 1. Relieving pain in childhood cancer

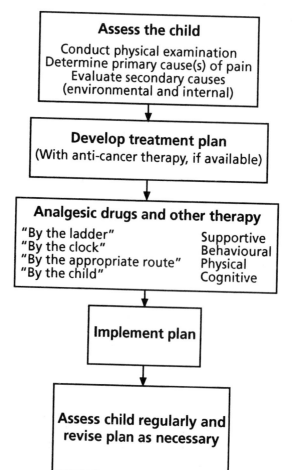

# Pain assessment

Pain assessment facilitates diagnosis and disease monitoring, and enables the health professional to alleviate needless suffering. The location, quality, severity, and duration of pain should be viewed as important clinical signs, since changes in a child's pain may signal a change in the disease process. This assessment should be continuous because the disease process and the factors that influence the attendant pain change over time. It must therefore include not only measurement of pain severity at a given point in time, but also an evaluation of how the various health-care, child, and family factors (see Fig. 1) may influence the pain. Responsibility for pain assessment should be shared by both health professionals and the child's family and caregivers.

The "ABCs" of pain assessment in children are:

- **Assess.** Always evaluate a child with cancer for potential pain. Children may experience pain, even though they may be unable to express the fact in words. Infants and toddlers can show their pain only by how they look and act; older children may deny their pain for fear of more painful treatment.

- **Body.** Be careful to consider pain as an integral part of the physical examination. Physical examination should include a comprehensive check of all body areas for potential pain sites. The child's reactions during the examination – grimacing, contracture, rigidity, etc. – may indicate pain.

- **Context.** Consider the impact of family, health-care, and environmental factors on the child's pain.

- **Document.** Record the severity of a child's pain on a regular basis. Use a pain scale that is simple and appropriate both for the developmental level of the child and for the cultural context in which it is used.

- **Evaluate.** Assess the effectiveness of pain interventions regularly and modify the treatment plan as necessary, until the child's pain is alleviated or minimized.

There are many ways to document pain severity that will provide an accurate, continuous record (7–11, 18). Some degree of pain assessment is always possible, even in the critically ill or cognitively impaired child. When children are unable to describe their pain in words, they must be carefully watched for behavioural signs of pain. Behavioural responses to pain may vary depending on whether the pain is brief or persistent; Table 2 outlines these differences. Many young children exhibit more obvious physical distress when a brief pain is strong. In contrast, children with persistent pain usually exhibit more subtle signs. Because parents and significant family members know their children and can recognize very subtle changes in manner or behaviour, they have a particularly important role in pain assessment. Behavioural signs, when present, can be helpful. However, absence of these signs does not necessarily mean absence of pain.

Table 2
**Primary behavioural signs indicative of pain in children**

| Behavioural signs | Duration of pain | |
| --- | --- | --- |
| | Brief | Persistent |
| Crying | + | |
| Distressed facial expression | + | |
| Motor disturbances (localized and whole body) | | + |
| Lack of interest in surroundings | | + |
| Decreased ability to concentrate | | + |
| Sleeping difficulties | | + |

Children under the age of 6 years can describe only the general amount of pain they feel, while older children can also describe other aspects – the severity, quality, location, duration, and changes over time. Pain severity can be determined by teaching children to use quantitative scales. Very simple scales with only two or three levels, such as pain "there" or "not there", or pain "small", "medium", and "large", can be adequate for assessing a child's pain. All such scales are based on the concept of counting, which is universal. Thus it is possible to develop practical tools for pain assessment that are appropriate for all cultures. When possible, a child should be asked "How strong is your pain now?"

He or she could answer by holding up a number of fingers, or in terms of the distance between their hands; pain severity could also be indicated by use of a tool, such as an abacus or a ruler.

The same system should be used to assess both the child's initial pain and the response to intervention. Pain should be recorded clearly on the child's clinical care chart and can be considered a vital sign. Appropriate pain-control therapies should be instituted and adjusted until there is a satisfactory response.

---

Optimal pain control begins with an accurate and thorough pain assessment.

A child's pain level is an essential vital sign and should be regularly recorded on the clinical record.

The severity of pain and the degree of relief should be considered as major factors in assessing quality of life and in weighing the benefits of additional curative or palliative therapies.

---

# Guidelines for non-drug pain relief therapy

Non-drug therapies must be an integral part of the management of children's cancer pain, beginning at the time of diagnosis and continuing throughout treatment. These therapies can be easily implemented in different settings and may substantially modify many of the factors that tend to increase pain. In some situations, non-drug therapy will activate sensory systems that block pain signals; in others it will trigger internal pain-inhibitory systems. Non-drug approaches should supplement, but not replace, appropriate drug treatment. They may be categorized as **supportive, cognitive, behavioural,** or **physical** ( *19*).

**Supportive** therapies support and empower the child and the family, **cognitive** therapies influence children's thoughts, **behavioural** therapies change behaviours, and **physical** therapies affect sensory systems. Most parents will intuitively use such approaches to relieve pain in their children – and children are usually aware that these methods can relieve pain. The following paragraphs describe how health care workers can help families to expand their use of these methods; see also the summary provided by Table 3.

## Supportive methods

Supportive methods are intended to promote the good psychosocial care of children. The first principle is that care is family- centred, that is, it is based on the needs of both family and child. Parental involvement in decision-making, and in providing comfort to children, is particularly important. Parents need a receptive environment and they may require instruction in how best to help their child. The importance of the family in ensuring the general health and well-being of children was recognized in a World Declaration on the Survival, Protection, and Development of Children at the World Summit for Children ( *20*):

> *The family has the primary responsibility for the nurturing and protection of children from infancy to adolescence ...*

*and all institutions of society should respect and support
the efforts of parents and other caregivers to nurture and
care for children in a family environment.*

The family includes everyone who is intimately associated with the child. In most cases it is the parents who know their children best and can therefore become allies in treatment, but they may need to be taught how they can help manage their children's pain and anxiety. Family-centred care encourages them to choose how to participate in treatment, giving them culturally appropriate information and teaching them coping techniques. It also helps family members to understand the cultural, spiritual, financial, social, interpersonal, and emotional impact of the diagnosis of cancer in a child.

Making the clinic or hospital environment friendly to families is another important aspect of family-centred care, and liberal visiting arrangements and a physical atmosphere conducive to family participation in treatment should be encouraged. It is essential that a child's family and friends are made to feel welcome.

Throughout the world, culturally-specific pain-reduction techniques or folk remedies are used and reflect the traditional wisdom, loyalties, and trust of the family, and the social sanctions of the community. It is important to respect such practices, to establish their compatibility with treatment, and to avoid alienating the family.

Both children and families need information to prepare them for what will happen during the course of the disease and its treatment. For example, it might help to explain a procedure to a child in the following way:

*We are going to put a needle in your back to get some fluid
that will help us understand how to help you best. You will
feel a cold spot on your back when we clean it. Then, a
pinch and some discomfort while we put in the numbing
medicine to make the nerves go to sleep. Then you will feel
some pressure while we push in the needle to get the fluid.
It should last about a minute. We will take out the needle
and put on a bandage and it shouldn't hurt any more.*

If families are not accurately informed about the diagnosis and the treatment plan, they cannot participate. Information is accepted best if it is tailored to the needs of the child and the family. Some children and families seek out information; others may find that too much information increases their anxiety. Health-care providers should therefore try to individualize their dealings with families. An empathic approach is essential, and information should be given a little at a time, repeated as frequently as needed. Booklets, videos, drawings, and dolls can be useful tools in this process.

Children should never be lied to about painful procedures; they will distrust and fear what will be done to them in the future. Health-care workers must be genuinely fond of children and know how to deal with them. Because of the multiple and complex demands placed on these caregivers, team leadership, support, and cohesion are essential to ensure the continuing quality of care. Ideally, children should be given choices about which techniques to use to control pain. They should also be allowed to make decisions that do not interfere with treatment, such as which finger to prick for blood samples.

Play is an essential part of every child's daily life and even the sickest child can be helped to play. Playing enables children to understand their world and to relax and forget their worries. All children must therefore have the time and place to play, and painful procedures must not be carried out in play areas. Normal activities such as school, hobbies, and visits by friends should be encouraged.

> Psychosocial treatment is an integral part of cancer pain treatment. It should be used in all painful or potentially painful situations, often combined with analgesic drug therapy.

## Cognitive methods

Cognitive treatment methods are intended to influence a child's thoughts and images. Parents are often very skilled at using these methods because they know their children's preferences. Active distraction of children's attention is important: the more involved a child becomes in an activity, the greater the distraction from pain. Infants and young children require concrete events or objects to attract their attention; interesting toys that provide something to see, hear, and do are best. Older children benefit from concentrating on a game, conversation, or special story. Music, even as simple as a mother's lullaby, is a universal soother and distractor (*21*). Children should be allowed their own choice of music.

**Imagery** (*22*) is the process in which a child concentrates on the image of a pleasant and interesting experience instead of on the pain. A child can be helped by an adult to become absorbed in a previous positive experience or an imaginary situation or adventure. Colours, sounds, tastes, smells, and atmosphere can all be experienced in imagination. Storytelling is a powerful way to engage the imagination and provide distraction; children may enjoy old favourites or new stories told from books or from memory.

**True hypnosis** (*23, 24*) requires specialized training, but pain can be modified by words of comfort and relief spoken in a particular way. Firstly, a child should be encouraged to relax and focus attention on a favourite activity, on deep breathing, or on a pain-free part of the body. Words such as the following may then be soothing:

> *Notice that the deeper you breathe, the more relaxed you feel. You may not feel the hurt as much as before. Notice how you feel more comfortable.*

Children can also imagine they are closing pain "switches" or "gates" or that they have the "magical" powers of their popular heroes to make their pain become less.

## Behavioural methods

**Deep breathing** is a simple way to help a child to reduce pain and gain self-control. It focuses the attention, reduces muscular tension, relaxes the diaphragm, and oxygenates the body. It is best to start teaching this technique by asking the child to breathe out, and to let go of the tension, or "scary" feelings, with each breath. Younger children can be taught to breathe deeply by blowing bubbles from soap solution or by using party blowers. Older children can use more sophisticated breathing techniques such as breathing in and out, each for the count of three.

**Progressive relaxation** – the sequential tensing and relaxing of muscle groups while lying down – is a useful technique for adolescents. Relaxation is often combined with suggestion and deep breathing, and these methods can reduce anticipatory anxiety and help to reduce nausea and vomiting.

## Physical methods

**Touch** is important for all children, particularly the pre-verbal child, who understands the world to a large extent through touching and feeling. Touch must be appropriate for the child's needs, that is, not too invasive either physically or psychologically. Touching includes stroking, holding and rocking, caressing, massaging hands, back, feet, head, and stomach, as well as swaddling. Vibration or tapping can also be comforting. When talking is too much effort for the child, touch can be the best form of communication. Cuddling combines several kinds of touch and is a comfort to most children.

When a child must be touched for medical purposes, e.g. palpation of the abdomen, care must be taken to use warm hands, to proceed gently, and to talk quietly with the child about what is being done.

Sources of heat and cold are often easily available (25). Ice wrapped in a cloth can be used to soothe disease pain or inflammation, or to reduce the pain of a procedure such as intramuscular injection. Ethyl chloride spray or "EMLA" cream (eutectic mixture of local anaesthetics; see page 54) offers a degree of anaesthesia at injection sites. Heat is useful for muscle pain. However, neither cold nor heat should be used on infants because there is a risk of injury.

**Transcutaneous electrical nerve stimulation** (TENS) is achieved with a battery-operated device that delivers electrical stimulation through electrodes placed on the skin. It possibly acts by cutaneous stimulation of large-diameter nerve fibres, reducing pain transmission at the spinal level. Children often experience TENS as tingling or tickling; it must not become painful. The technique is simple to use, is effective, and requires little preparation (26). Children themselves and their families can often use TENS after simple instruction and explanation.

Table 3
**Non-drug methods of pain relief**

| Supportive | Cognitive | Behavioural | Physical |
|---|---|---|---|
| Family-centred care Information Empathy Choices Play | Distraction Music Imagery Hypnosis | Deep breathing Relaxation | Touch Heat and cold[a] Transcutaneous electrical nerve stimulation (TENS) |

[a] Heat and cold should not be used with infants because of the risk of injury.

## Case example: non-drug therapy

A 3-year-old boy with acute lymphocytic leukaemia requires intravenous vincristine therapy. Previously, he cried and had to be held down when intravenous treatments were started; now he is whimpering and clinging to his mother. His mother is anxious but cooperative. She has explained to him in a way he can understand what will happen and how it will feel. In the waiting room he is given some soap solution and a wire loop for blowing bubbles. His mother shows him how to make the bubbles. The boy enjoys this and plays while the intravenous line is being prepared. Mother and child then go into the treatment room and the boy continues to blow bubbles while the injection site is prepared and the tourniquet is applied. He chooses to sit on his mother's lap during the procedure and is encouraged to "blow away the hurt" as the needle is inserted. His mother and all the medical staff praise him for being brave. When he tires of blowing bubbles, his mother reads him his favourite story.

# Guidelines for analgesic drug therapy

The non-drug approaches outlined above target all causes of pain – physical and psychological – and should be an integral part of all interventions designed to control pain in childhood cancer. However, the optimal approach to cancer pain management in children includes drug therapy, with analgesic drugs usually considered the mainstay of treatment. Correct use of analgesic drugs will relieve pain in most children and relies on the following four key concepts:

- "by the ladder"
- "by the clock"
- "by the appropriate route"
- "by the child".

## "By the ladder"

A three-step approach to analgesia, described as an analgesic "ladder", has repeatedly been shown to be effective; it is illustrated in Fig. 2. Pain is classified as mild, moderate, or severe, and analgesic choices are adjusted accordingly. The ladder approach is based on drugs that are widely available in most countries and relies on physicians and health professionals knowing how to make the best use of a limited number of drugs. Paracetamol, codeine, and morphine are the recommended analgesics for cancer pain in children, but alternatives may be substituted if these are unavailable or not well tolerated. Dosage recommendations are given in the section *Specific drugs for pain relief.*

The sequential use of analgesic drugs is based on the child's level of pain, and the first step in controlling mild pain is a non-opioid analgesic. Paracetamol is the drug of choice for children who can take oral medication. If pain persists, an opioid for mild to moderate pain should be given; codeine is the drug of choice for this purpose. Children should continue to receive paracetamol – or a non-steroidal anti-inflammatory drug (NSAID) if appropriate — for supplementary analgesia. When an opioid for mild to moderate pain combined with a non-opioid fails to provide relief, an opioid for moderate to severe pain should be substituted; again, paracetamol (or NSAID if appropriate) should be continued. Morphine is the drug of choice in this instance. Adjuvant drugs may be given for specific indications.

There should be no hesitation in moving up to the next step of the analgesic ladder if pain control is inadequate, but only one drug from each of the groups should be used at the same time. If a drug (e.g. codeine) ceases to be effective, a drug that is *definitely stronger* (e.g. morphine) should be prescribed, rather than an alternative drug of similar efficacy. When an opioid for moderate to severe pain is used, its dose may be increased until pain is relieved or there are signs of toxicity; an alternative drug from the same category should then be substituted.

**Fig. 2. The three-step analgesic ladder**

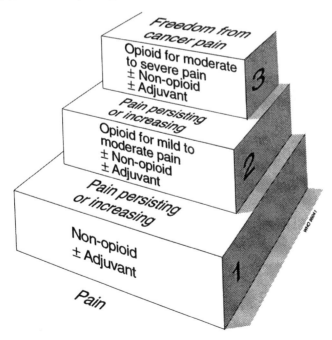

## "By the clock"

Medication should be administered according to a regular schedule, i.e. "by the clock", rather than on a *pro re nata* (prn) or as-required basis, unless pain episodes are truly intermittent and unpredictable. On a prn basis, children must experience pain before they are able to obtain medication; they may fear that their pain cannot be controlled and so become increasingly frightened. In addition, the doses of opioids required to prevent the recurrence of pain are lower than those required to treat episodic pain. Children should therefore receive analgesics at regular intervals, with additional "rescue" doses for intermittent and breakthrough pain. The dosing interval should be determined according to the severity of the pain and the duration of action of the drug in question.

## "By the appropriate route"

Drugs should be administered to children by the simplest, most effective, and least painful route. Analgesics are usually given orally in the form of tablets and elixirs. Intravenous, subcutaneous, and transdermal administration may also be appropriate. The advantages and disadvantages of the different routes of administration are shown in Table 4.

In general, intramuscular injections should not be used unless absolutely necessary; they are painful and thus frightening to children who may respond by failing to request pain medication or by denying that they have pain. Rectal administration is unpleasant for many children but it is preferable to intramuscular administration. If injections are necessary, a eutectic mixture of 2.5% lidocaine and 2.5% prilocaine in the form of a cream (or other topical formulation of lidocaine) helps to reduce the pain caused by needles (*27*).

Patient-controlled analgesia (PCA) is a novel approach to intravenous or subcutaneous administration of drugs; it allows children over about 7 years of age to push a button to give themselves "rescue" doses of analgesics for breakthrough pain. A pre-set dose is delivered into an infusion line by a computer-driven pump. For safety, there is a timed lock-out period after each dose so that additional doses cannot be delivered before a specified time has elapsed. PCA may be used alone or with concurrent continuous infusions (*9, 28*).

Table 4

**Routes of drug administration: advantages and disadvantages**

| Oral | Transdermal | Intravenous | Sub-cutaneous | Intramuscular | Rectal |
|------|-------------|-------------|---------------|---------------|--------|
| • Painless<br>• Preferred by children | • Painless<br>• Restricted to fentanyl: contraindicated in opioid-naive patients<br>• Not indicated for acute pain management<br>• Not indicated for escalating pain<br>• Can be used if pain has been stabilized | • Rapid pain control<br>• Easiest to titrate and to adjust to rapidly changing pain levels<br>• Useful for intermittent bolus and continuous infusion<br>• Appropriate for PCA[a] | • Avoids need for IV line<br>• Useful for home setting<br>• Useful for continuous infusion<br>• Appropriate for PCA[a] | • Painful<br>• Not recommended<br>• Wide variability in therapeutic blood levels | • Generally disliked by children<br>• Wide variability in therapeutic blood levels<br>• Variable absorption<br>• Can be used if there is transient vomiting |

[a] PCA = patient-controlled analgesia

27

Considerations in selecting the best route of analgesic administration for children with cancer pain include the severity of the pain, the type of pain, the potency of the drug, and the required dosing interval.

## "By the child"

Doses of all medications must be based upon each child's circumstances: there is no single dose that will be appropriate for all children. The goal is to select a dose that prevents the child from experiencing pain before the next dose is due to be administered. It is essential to monitor the child's pain regularly and to adjust analgesic doses as necessary to control it. The opioid dose that effectively relieves pain varies widely between children and in the same child at different times, and should therefore be based on the individual child's pain level. Very large opioid doses are needed at frequent intervals to control pain in some children; provided that the side-effects are minimal or can be managed by adjunctive medication, these doses may be regarded as appropriate. Children receiving opioids may develop altered sleep patterns, becoming wakeful at night, fearful, and complaining about pain, and sleeping intermittently during the day. Adequate analgesics should be given at night, together with hypnotics or antidepressants as necessary, to enable such children to sleep throughout the night. To relieve severe, continuing pain, opioid doses should be increased steadily until comfort is achieved, unless there are unacceptable side-effects such as somnolence and respiratory depression, in which case an alternative opioid should be tried. Incomplete cross-tolerance between various opioids may mean that another opioid will be effective at a lower dose and with minimal side-effects.

# Specific drugs for pain relief

## Non-opioid analgesics

Non-opioid analgesics are used to relieve mild pain or, in combination with opioids, to relieve moderate and severe pain (*29*). All have analgesic, antipyretic, and − except for paracetamol − anti-inflammatory effects. Paracetamol is the drug of choice because it has a very high therapeutic ratio for children. The recommended dose is 10–15 mg/kg orally every 4–6 hours. Unlike acetylsalicylic acid (aspirin), paracetamol has no gastrointestinal or haematological side-effects and lacks the possible association with Reye syndrome. Moreover, newborns and young infants tolerate paracetamol without difficulty. The use of acetylsalicylic acid and other NSAIDs is more restricted in children than in adults with cancer because of potential bleeding problems; this is a major concern, as children with cancer often have very low platelet counts. However, NSAIDs are useful for children with bone metastases, provided that platelet counts are adequate, but they should be used with caution in newborns. Ibuprofen (10 mg/kg orally, every 6–8 hours) is an example and is included in the WHO *Model List of Essential Drugs*.[1] Alternatives include naproxen (5 mg/kg orally, every 8–12 hours) and tolmetin (5–10 mg/kg orally every 6-8 hours). Since all of these drugs can cause gastritis, they should be administered with meals. Choline magnesium trisalicylate (10–15 mg/kg orally, every 8–12 hours) causes relatively little gastritis, but shares with aspirin the disadvantage of an association with Reye syndrome.

Increasing the dose of non-opioid analgesics beyond the recommended therapeutic level (Table 5) produces a "ceiling" effect, in that there is little additional analgesia but a significant increase in side-effects and toxic reactions. If a non-opioid, with or without an adjuvant drug, fails to provide adequate relief of mild to moderate pain, an opioid for mild to moderate pain should be added. If the pain is severe, an opioid for moderate to severe pain should be added.

---

[1]  *The use of essential drugs: eighth report of the WHO Expert Committee*. Geneva, World Health Organization, 1998 (WHO Technical Report Series, No. 882).

Table 5
**Non-opioid drugs for relieving cancer pain in children**

| Drug | Dosage | Remarks |
|------|--------|---------|
| Paracetamol | 10–15 mg/kg orally, every 4–6 hours | Has no gastrointestinal or haematological side-effects, but lacks anti-inflammatory activity |
| Ibuprofen | 5–10 mg/kg orally, every 6–8 hours | Anti-inflammatory activity, but may have gastrointestinal and haematological side-effects |
| Naproxen | 5 mg/kg orally, every 8–12 hours | Anti-inflammatory activity, but may have gastrointestinal and haematological side-effects |

## Opioid analgesics for mild to moderate pain

Codeine is the opioid of choice for mild to moderate cancer pain in children. The recommended starting dose is 0.5–1.0 mg/kg orally every 3–4 hours for children over 6 months of age. As with stronger opioids, the starting dose of codeine for infants less than 6 months old should be between one-quarter and one-third of the dose (mg/kg) for older children. Codeine is usually administered in fixed combinations with non-opioids (usually paracetamol). Parenteral administration is not recommended. If no pain relief is achieved at the recommended dose, codeine should be discontinued and a stronger opioid administered: doses above the recommended level may increase side-effects without greatly improving analgesia. Dosage guidelines are summarized in Table 6.

## Opioid analgesics for moderate to severe pain

Strong opioid analgesics are required to relieve severe cancer pain. These drugs are simple to administer and provide effective pain relief in the majority of children (*9, 15, 16, 30*). They can be used alone or in combination with non-opioid analgesics and/or adjuvant drugs, depending on the sources of pain; for example, pain relief can be enhanced by continuing the use of an NSAID or paracetamol in addition to an opioid.

The safe, rational use of opioid analgesics requires an understanding of their clinical pharmacology. Strong opioids have no fixed upper dosage limit because there is no analgesic "ceiling" effect. The right dose is the dose that provides satisfactory relief of pain. Children may require extremely large doses to obtain relief, sometimes as much as a thousand times the standard starting dose. The need for an increasing dose to maintain adequate pain control may result from spread of the disease or from increased drug tolerance, and children should be carefully evaluated for progression of disease before drug tolerance is assumed. Opioid treatment for more than 7 days will cause physio-logical dependence and should be discontinued only by a gradual tapering of dosage to avoid the symptoms of withdrawal. A typical tapering regimen might be a 50% reduction of the dose for 2 days followed by a 25% reduction every 2 days until the opioid dose is equianalgesic to an oral morphine dose of 0.6 mg/kg per day for a child weighing less than 50 kg or 30 mg/day for a child over 50 kg. When that point is reached, the drug can be discontinued.

Side-effects of opioids such as constipation, itching, and sedation are common, and they should be anticipated and treated aggressively. Parents should be advised that there may be some sedation with initial dosing, but that this generally abates within a few days. If not prepared for this, parents often worry unnecessarily that somnolence indicates that the disease is progressing and that their child may be dying.

Initial opioid dosage should also be reduced in children with severe malnutrition, hepatic or renal dysfunction, or multi-organ failure, or in whom there is pre-existing sedation.

> Non-opioid analgesics have a "ceiling" effect. Opioid drugs do not.
> The correct dose of opioid is the dose that provides adequate
> relief of pain with an acceptable degree of side-effects.

The strong opioid of choice included in WHO's *Model List of Essential Drugs* is morphine.[1] Alternatives are hydromorphone, methadone, and fentanyl. Pethidine is not recommended for chronic use because of accumulation of the toxic metabolite norpethidine.

Dosage guidelines are summarized in Table 6.

---

[1] *The use of essential drugs: eighth report of the WHO Expert Committee.* Geneva, World Health Organization, 1998 (WHO Technical Report Series, No. 882).

Table 6
**Opioid analgesic dosage guidelines for opioid-naive patients**

| Opioid | Equianalgesic doses[a] | | Usual IV or SC starting dose[b] | | Parenteral:oral dose ratio | Usual oral starting dose[b] | | Biological half-life (hours) |
|---|---|---|---|---|---|---|---|---|
| | Parenteral | Oral | Child <50 kg | Child ≥50 kg | | Child <50 kg | Child ≥50 kg | |
| *Short half-life opioids* | | | | | | | | |
| Codeine | 130 mg | 200 mg | N/R[c] | N/R[c] | 1:1.5 | 0.5–1 mg/kg every 3–4 hours | 30 mg every 3–4 hours | 2.5–3 |
| Oxycodone | N/A[d] | 30 mg | N/A[d] | N/A[d] | N/A[d] | 0.2 mg/kg every 3–4 hours | 5–10 mg every 3–4 hours | 2–3 |
| Pethidine[e] N/R[c] | 75 mg N/R[c] | 300 mg N/R[c] | 0.75 mg/kg every 2–4 hours N/R[c] | 75–100 mg every 2–4 hours N/R[c] | 1:4 | 1–1.5 mg/kg every 3–4 hours N/R[c] | 50–75 mg every 3–4 hours N/R[c] | 3 |
| Morphine | 10 mg | 30 mg | Bolus dose: 0.05–0.1 mg/kg IV or SC every 2–4 hours Continuous infusion: 0.03 mg/kg per hour | 5–10 mg IV or SC every 2–4 hours Continuous infusion: 1 mg/hour | 1:3 | 0.15–0.3 mg/kg every 4 hours | 5–10 mg every 4 hours | 2.5–3 |
| Hydromorphone | 1.5 mg | 7.5 mg | 0.015 mg/kg every 2–4 hours | 1–1.5 mg/kg every 2–4 hours | 1:5 | 0.06 mg/kg every 3–4 hours | 2 mg every 3–4 hours | 2–3 |
| Oxymorphone | 1 mg | N/A[d] | 0.02 mg/kg every 2–4 hours | 1 mg every 2–4 hours | N/A[d] | N/A[d] | N/A[d] | 1.5 |

*WORLD HEALTH ORGANIZATION*

# CANCER PAIN RELIEF AND PALLIATIVE CARE IN CHILDREN

## CORRIGENDUM

Page 32, Table 6

Under "Usual IV or SC starting dose", the dose of hydromorphone for a child ⩾ 50 kg should read:

**1–1.5 mg every 2–4 hours**

| Opioid | Equianalgesic doses[a] | | Usual IV or SC starting dose[b] | | Parenteral:oral dose ratio | Usual oral starting dose[b] | | Biological half-life (hours) |
| --- | --- | --- | --- | --- | --- | --- | --- | --- |
| | Parenteral | Oral | Child <50 kg | Child ≥50 kg | | Child <50 kg | Child ≥50 kg | |
| Fentanyl[f] | 100 µg single dose | N/A[d] | 0.5–2 µg/kg per hour as continuous infusion | 25–75 µg every 1 hour | N/A[d] | N/A[d] | N/A[d] | 3 |
| **Long half-life opioids** | | | | | | | | |
| Controlled-release morphine | N/A[d] | N/A[d] | N/A[d] | N/A[d] | N/A[d] | 0.6 mg/kg every 8 hours, *or* 0.9 mg/kg every 12 hours | 30–60 mg every 12 hours | |
| Methadone[g] | 10 mg | 20 mg | 0.1 mg/kg IV or SC every 4–8 hours | 5–10 mg IV or SC every 4–8 hours | 1:2 | 0.2 mg/kg every 4–8 hours | 5–10 mg every 4–8 hours | 12–50 |

a   Equianalgesic doses are based on single-dose studies in adults.
b   Usual starting dose is the commonly used standard dose and not always based on equianalgesic principles (i.e. starting dose of hydromorphone may be 2 mg despite the parenteral:oral ratio of 1:5). For infants under 6 months of age, starting doses should be one-quarter to one-third the suggested dose and titrated to effect.
c   N/R = not recommended.
d   N/A = not applicable.
e   Pethidine is not recommended for chronic use because of its long half-life and the possibility of accumulation of a toxic metabolite.
f   Continuous infusion of fentanyl at 100 µg/hour is approximately equianalgesic to a morphine infusion of 2.5 mg/hour.
g   Methadone may cause some irritation when administered SC. Extreme care is needed when using methadone, both for initiation of therapy and when doses are increased, because of the extremely long biological half-life (see page 38).

*Important notes*

1.   For all drugs for which a distinction is made between children <50 kg and those ≥50 kg, doses should be calculated in mg/kg for children <50 kg and the "usual adult dose" should be used for those ≥50 kg.
2.   When a change is made to short-half-life opioids in an opioid-tolerant patient, the new drug should be given at 50% of the equianalgesic dose (because of incomplete cross-tolerance) and titrated to effect.

33

## Morphine

Morphine is the drug of choice for controlling severe pain for most children (*31–33*) and is the standard against which the analgesic properties of other drugs are measured. The recommended starting dose is 0.15–0.3 mg/kg orally, every 4 hours, titrated individually until the pain is relieved. Oral preparations of morphine sulfate and morphine hydrochloride are available. The aqueous solutions are bitter, so children prefer the drug mixed in a flavoured syrup. Morphine solution should be stored in a dark bottle, out of direct sunlight, and in a cool place; an antimicrobial preservative is necessary, particularly in warmer climates.

The pharmacokinetics of morphine in young infants are different from those in older children; consequently, initial opioid dosage (on a mg/kg basis) in infants less than 6 months of age should be between one-quarter and one-third of the initial dose for older children. Opioids should be administered to infants in a setting where continuous observation and immediate intervention are possible in case of delayed respiratory depression developing as a side-effect.

If oral administration is not possible, continuous intravenous (IV) or subcutaneous (SC) infusion starting at 0.03 mg/kg per hour is effective in producing a constant analgesic effect. Alternatively, intermittent doses starting at 0.05–0.1 mg/kg can be given every 2–4 hours through an indwelling SC or IV line. During long-term administration, the oral dose of morphine (in mg/kg) should be approximately three times the parenteral dose.

If prolonged pain is anticipated, controlled-release oral morphine preparations are valuable. These may be given at intervals of 8–12 hours and, because fewer daily doses are required, children can sleep without interruption. Tablets vary in strength from 10 to 200 mg, but are not available in all countries. It should be noted that the controlled-release properties are destroyed by crushing the tablets. However, controlled-release "sprinkles" or "beads" are available in some countries; these formulations do not lose their controlled-release properties when the capsules in which they are contained are opened. The recommended starting dose is 0.6 mg/kg every 8 hours or 0.9 mg/kg every 12 hours. This preparation is more difficult to titrate to effect than regular morphine. To titrate the correct dosage, regular oral morphine should be given every 4 hours, and the dose should be titrated to achieve pain control throughout a 24-hour period. The controlled-release preparation should then be substituted; 100% of the total 24-hour dose of oral morphine that provided effective pain relief should be administered, either as three 8-hourly doses or as two 12-hourly doses.

Common dosing considerations for administering morphine to children are summarized in the following case examples:

### Case example: initial intravenous morphine titration and oral conversion

A 2-year-old boy, weighing 12 kg, has severe pain.

- Initial intravenous morphine titration:
  - Starting dose of morphine 0.1 mg/kg x 12 kg = 1.2 mg.
  - Reassess in 30 minutes.
  - If child is still in pain and not sedated, repeat dose of 1.2 mg.
  - If child is still in pain but somewhat sedated, give 25–50% of starting dose (0.3–0.6 mg).
  - The child is now comfortable.

- Continuous infusion of morphine:
  - Start morphine infusion at dose of (0.03 mg/kg per hour) x 12 kg = 0.36 mg/hour (i.e. approximately 0.4 mg/hour). Provide hourly rescue doses for breakthrough pain at 50–200% of hourly infusion dose, i.e. 0.2–0.8 mg.
  - Assess in 1 hour. Child is still comfortable.
  - Reassess after 4 hours. Child has moderate pain; he is withdrawn and cries when not held.

- Titration:
  - Administer rescue bolus. If repeated breakthrough pain occurs, increase infusion dose by 25% (0.25 x 0.36 = 0.09 mg), i.e. increase to 0.36 + 0.09 = 0.45 mg/hour. Continue to provide rescue doses.
  - Alternatively, continue with rescue doses for 24 hours, then increase the infusion by the amount of morphine administered in rescue doses. For example, if six rescue doses of 0.5 mg were given, increase hourly infusion rate by (6 x 0.5 mg)/24 hours =

0.12 mg; the new infusion rate thus becomes 0.36 + 0.12 = approximately 0.48 mg/hour.

— Alternatively, a 4-hourly subcutaneous dose could be given, with hourly rescue doses.

- Oral conversion:

  — Next morning, the child is still comfortable and gets up to play. Calculate the total 24-hour intravenous dose (24 x 0.48 = 11.5 mg). Since the oral:parenteral ratio is 3:1, the equivalent oral dose is 3 x 11.5 = 34.5 mg (or approximately 35 mg). Continue with 4-hourly oral morphine at a dose of 6 mg (35 mg/6 = approximately 6 mg).

  — Alternatively, if controlled-release preparations (35 mg/2 or 35 mg/3) are available, give 15 mg every 12 hours or 12 mg every 8 hours.

  — For breakthrough pain give a dose of immediate-release morphine, at 5–10% of the child's 24-hour opioid dose (0.1 x 35 = 3.5 mg, or approximately 4 mg), as needed, in addition to regular scheduled doses.

## Case example: management of night-time breakthrough pain

An 8-year-old boy with chronic pain is comfortable at home on a stable oral dose of 30 mg morphine every 4 hours. He takes his 22:00 dose and goes to sleep; at 03.00 he wakes in pain and is given another oral dose of morphine.

- Change dosing pattern to help the child sleep pain-free. Increase the bedtime (22:00) dose by 50%, i.e. give 45 mg morphine.

- Alternatively, change the dosage form to controlled-release morphine. Since 30 mg every 4 hours is a daily total of 180 mg, change to 90 mg controlled-release morphine every 12 hours or 60 mg controlled-release morphine every 8 hours. Continue to provide rescue doses.

- Alternatively, wake the child at 02:00 to give him the 30-mg oral dose.

## Case example: respiratory depression and somnolence due to oral morphine elixir

A 1-year-old baby girl, weighing 10 kg, has moderate to severe retroperitoneal pain from recently diagnosed metastatic neuroblastoma; she is fussy and difficult to console. Her starting respiration rate is 35/minute.

- A strong opioid is indicated for moderate to severe pain, given orally or parenterally. For rapid pain relief and for purposes of titration, intravenous administration of 0.1 mg/kg morphine would be preferable, but the oral route (which would permit treatment at home) is chosen. The oral:parenteral ratio is 3:1; an oral dose of 0.3 mg/kg x 10 kg = 3 mg is therefore administered at 06:00 and repeated every 4 hours.

- At 07:00 the baby is free of pain.

- At 18:00, after three doses, the baby becomes (and remains) sleepy; her breathing is shallow and her respiration rate 10/minute.

- Stimulate the baby immediately and administer oxygen. Check oxygen saturation if facilities are available. Continue to monitor her condition carefully.

- At 22:00, withhold the next dose of morphine and allow the baby to become more alert and active, with deeper breathing, a normal respiration rate, and oxygen saturation >95%.

- Reduce subsequent doses of morphine by 50%, i.e. give 1.5 mg every 4 hours.

- The baby remains comfortable but alert with continued morphine dosing at this reduced level.

## Hydromorphone

Hydromorphone is similar to morphine in its pharmacokinetics, efficacy, and toxicity, but it is about six times more potent on parenteral administration and eight times more potent when given orally. It is available for oral, rectal, and parenteral administration, and its oral:parenteral ratio is 5:1. The oral elixir may be more palatable for children than morphine elixir. Hydromorphone is also available in a high-potency formulation (10 mg/ml and in some countries 50 mg/ml), suitable for SC infusion when high doses in small volumes are required. When morphine is contraindicated or produces unacceptable side-effects, hydromorphone is a useful alternative opioid.

## Methadone

Methadone is a synthetic, long-acting opioid analgesic, which is recommended for children unable to tolerate morphine and hydro-morphone because of side-effects (e.g. nausea and sedation). The prolonged half-life of methadone necessitates extremely careful dosage adjustments to achieve pain control. A starting oral dose of 0.2 mg/kg is recommended, but effective dosing intervals may range from 4 to 12 hours (see case example below). Although a child may appear to tolerate methadone well for the first few days, accumulation of the drug may slowly occur, leading to signs of overdosage during the subsequent few days. Thus where other strong opioids are administered by the clock, methadone should initially be given 4-hourly *as required*. Any child given methadone should be carefully monitored for several days after the drug is initiated and whenever the dose is increased. After 24–48 hours, when the child's requirement is well established, round-the-clock dosing can be initiated. If somnolence or shallow breathing occurs, the methadone should be withheld until the child is awake and the breathing pattern normalizes; methadone administration can then be resumed at 50% of the previous dose or at longer dosing intervals.

The oral route of administration is preferable; if parenteral administration is required, approximately 50% of the oral dose will effectively control pain in most children. Children who are severely debilitated or who have significant impairment of hepatic or renal function should be given lower doses initially, which can then be increased as required. As with morphine, the dose can be increased to the level necessary to achieve pain relief, as long as children do not suffer dose-limiting side-effects.

Methadone and other long-acting opioids should be used with extreme caution in children with rapidly changing clinical conditions or with metabolic complications that may suddenly affect drug clearance and intensify side-effects. Drugs with shorter half-lives should be used in most circumstances.

### Case example: methadone dosing (oral elixir)

A 2-year-old child, weighing 14 kg, with widespread tumour, has severe pain. Oral hydromorphone has been stopped because she suffered unacceptable side-effects (as she had previously had with morphine). Her baseline respiratory rate is 32/minute.

- First dose of methadone, 0.2 mg/kg x 14 kg = 2.8 mg, is given orally at 07:00:

    - After 1 hour, the child's pain has been relieved.

— At 11:00 the child has moderate pain. The 2.8 mg dose is repeated and good analgesia is achieved.

- Recommended dosing:
  — Methadone should be given on an as-required basis for the first 2–3 days; the maintenance dose and dosing interval should then be calculated according to the most recent requirements.
  — For this child, dosing should be continued at 2.8 mg every 6–8 hours, with regular assessment.

- The clinician continues to give the child the recommended methadone dose, but fails to assess her condition regularly. The child remains comfortable for 2 days but becomes very sleepy on the third day, with shallow respiration at a rate of 10/minute:
  — Withhold the methadone until the child is easily aroused and her respiration improves.
  — Subsequently, reduce the dose by 50% (i.e. to 1.4 mg) or lengthen the dosing interval to 8–12 hours.

## Fentanyl

Fentanyl is a synthetic opioid that is shorter-acting than morphine when administered as a single bolus. It can be used to relieve severe pain caused by brief invasive procedures and as an infusion for continuous pain. The IV dose for brief procedures is 1–2 µg/kg 5 minutes before the procedure. For infusion, the recommended starting dose is 1–2 µg/kg per hour IV. Fentanyl causes less histamine release than morphine, so it is also useful for pain in children who have severe pruritus, resistant to treatment with antihistamines. Rapid administration of >3 µg/kg may produce chest wall rigidity and severe ventilatory difficulty. This complication is reversible with the opioid antagonist naloxone. Sufentanil and alfentanil, analogues of fentanyl with even shorter durations of action, may be especially useful to control pain during short invasive procedures.

Fentanyl is also available in a patch form for transdermal absorption. In this form it is of no value for acute pain, and it is not indicated in opiate-naive patients or in situations where the dose for effective pain relief is still being titrated. The time from application to peak effect is approximately 12-16 hours and the drug has an elimination half-life of 21 hours. Fentanyl patches are used for management of chronic pain in children over 12 years of age and over 50 kg in weight.

# Treatment of opioid side-effects

All opioid drugs cause similar side-effects. These problems are well known and should be anticipated and treated whenever children are given opioids, so that pain control is not accompanied by unacceptable side-effects. Children often do not voluntarily report all side-effects (e.g. constipation, dysphoria, pruritus), so they should be asked specific questions about these problems. Some side-effects – nausea, vomiting, and somnolence, for example – may resolve within the first week of initiating therapy, but others will require aggressive treatment. If side-effects persist despite appropriate interventions, a different opioid should be tried, whose side-effects may be better tolerated. There is generally incomplete cross-tolerance of opioids, so that when one opioid is substituted for another, the new drug should be started at 50% of the equianalgesic dose and titrated to establish the effective dose.

## Constipation

Constipation is an expected side-effect of opioid administration and does not resolve. It can be avoided by giving a suitable diet (increased fluids and bulk) and by the daily administration of stool softeners, such as docusate, combined with a stimulant, such as senna.

## Nausea and/or vomiting

When opioids are the cause of nausea and/or vomiting, an antiemetic such as metoclopramide (0.1–0.2 mg/kg IV or orally every 6 hours to a maximum of 15 mg per dose) or a phenothiazine such as prochlorperazine (0.1–0.2 mg/kg IV or orally every 6 hours to a maximum of 10 mg per dose) may be given. In a small number of cases these drugs can cause extrapyramidal side-effects, such as dystonia. Dystonia can be treated with an antihistamine, usually given parenterally for rapid effect. Diphenhydramine (0.5–1 mg/kg IV or orally to a maximum of 50 mg per dose) is appropriate. Antihistamines such as diphenhydramine or hydroxyzine can also be used as antiemetics at a dose of 0.5–1 mg/kg orally or IV (slowly and through a central line for hydroxyzine) every 4–6 hours to a maximum of 50 mg per dose.

## Pruritus

The antihistamines diphenhydramine and hydroxyzine can be used as specified above to treat opioid-related itching. It may also be appropriate to change the opioid to fentanyl or oxymorphone; these drugs cause less histamine release and may produce fewer or less severe side-effects.

## Respiratory depression

When respiratory depression occurs, management should be based on the child's specific health status and treatment goals. If the child is terminally ill, for example, respiratory compromise is part of the dying process and attempts to treat the problem may not always be appropriate if they would intensify or prolong suffering.

When respiratory depression is mild and reversal is appropriate, simple methods are often effective. These include stimulating the child, reminding him or her to breathe, and withholding the next dose of opioid. Subsequent opioid dosing should be reduced by 50% initially and then titrated to maintain pain relief without respiratory depression.

Pharmacological reversal with an opioid antagonist is rarely required. For severe respiratory depression, however, airway support should be maintained, supplemental oxygen provided, and naloxone administered to the point of reversal of respiratory depression without compromising pain relief, if possible. Naloxone should be titrated carefully (generally increments of 0.5–2 µg/kg or 20 µg IV every 1–2 minutes). The greater the tolerance of the child to opioids, the greater will be the sensitivity to the effects of naloxone, and there is a risk of profound distress caused by withdrawal symptoms. Thus in the opioid-tolerant patient naloxone must be titrated by very small amounts to avoid precipitating withdrawal, which is extremely distressing and potentially dangerous. Children must be continually monitored following treatment with naloxone because the effects of opioids last longer than those of the antagonist – the half-life of naloxone is much shorter than that of any of the opioids.

## Confusion and/or hallucinations

There are many causes of central nervous system side-effects in children with cancer. If careful investigation reveals that confusion and/or hallucinations are clearly opioid-related, the opioid should be changed or a neuroleptic such as haloperidol (0.01–0.1 mg/kg orally or IV every 8 hours to a maximum dose of 30 mg/day) should be added. Neuroleptics should be used with caution because of the potential for extrapyramidal side-effects.

## Myoclonus

Myoclonus is a sudden, involuntary jerking movement of the extremities, head, or trunk, which is considered "benign" if it occurs around the time of sleep. If myoclonus is present during waking hours or is severe, a benzodiazepine can be given (e.g. clonazepam, starting with 0.01 mg/kg orally every 12 hours to a maximum of 0.5 mg per dose) or the opioid can be changed.

## Somnolence

If somnolence fails to resolve within a week of starting opioids, and if the child and/or family find it disturbing, a psychostimulant such as dexamfetamine (dexamphetamine) or methylphenidate can be given (0.1 mg/kg twice daily, in the morning and at midday so as not to interfere with night-time sleep). The dose can be raised in increments of 0.05–0.1 mg/kg to a maximum of 0.5 mg/kg per day.

# Opioid dependence and tolerance

Fear of what is commonly thought of as opioid addiction is one of the principal reasons for children with severe cancer pain not receiving adequate analgesia. This fear has been greatly exaggerated. "Addiction" occurs when individuals are overwhelmingly involved in obtaining and using a drug primarily for its euphoric effects. This is not a problem in children with cancer who receive opioids for pain control.

Physical dependence and tolerance are physiological phenomena, however, and occur in everyone taking opioids on a chronic basis. Physiological (physical) dependence occurs when the body becomes accustomed to a certain level of drug and therefore requires the drug on a continuous basis. If opioids are suddenly withdrawn, children suffer irritability, anxiety, insomnia, diaphoresis, rhinorrhoea, nausea, vomiting, abdominal cramps, and diarrhoea. If opioids are no longer required for pain control, withdrawal symptoms can be avoided in children who have been on opioid therapy for longer than a week by gradual tapering of doses.

Tolerance to opioid drugs occurs after repeated administration; there is gradual adjustment to a certain drug level and progressively higher doses of opioids become necessary to achieve the same degree of pain relief. Although children with cancer pain may require increasing and more frequent opioid doses because of tolerance, they should receive the doses necessary to relieve their pain. Nevertheless, whenever increased opioid doses are needed to relieve previously controlled pain, children should also be assessed carefully to determine whether the disease has progressed, since pain may be the first sign of advancing disease.

Parents are often anxious about opioid use for their children, particularly when they require increasing doses. It is therefore essential for health-care workers to reassure families that opioid dependence and tolerance are normal phenomena and do not mean that a child has become "addicted". Children and adolescents may also manifest "drug-seeking behaviour", such as making frequent demands for opioids, requesting increasing doses, and "watching the clock". This behaviour pattern – "pseudo-addiction" – is often seen when pain management is sub-optimal and generally resolves once the problem is aggressively addressed and the medication titrated to provide satisfactory relief.

# Adjuvant therapy

Many drugs can relieve the symptoms experienced by children with cancer. So-called "adjuvant drugs" may help to relieve pain by elevating mood, reducing anxiety levels, or minimizing the adverse side-effects of the primary analgesic drugs, or by enhancing analgesia directly. Unlike opioid and non-opioid analgesics, use of adjuvant drugs for pain control and symptom relief in children is generally based on uncontrolled trials and anecdotal clinical experience. Adjuvant drugs should not be prescribed routinely: their role in cancer pain management should be based on the needs of each child. Continual reassessment of the indications for, and the efficacy of, adjuvant drugs should guide their acute or chronic use in children. Table 7 summarizes the major adjuvant drug groups, which are discussed in more detail in the following sections.

## Antidepressants

Tricyclic antidepressants can relieve pain as well as depression. They are the drugs of choice to alleviate neuropathic pain (burning pain resulting from nerve damage or inflammation, such as vincristine-induced neuropathy, tumour invasion, or nerve resection). Tricyclic antidepressants also improve sleep and can enhance opioid analgesia. An initial oral dose of 0.2–0.5 mg/kg of amitriptyline, with a maximum starting dose of 25 mg, is recommended at bedtime, increasing by 25% every 2–3 days to antidepressant levels, if needed. Usually, sleep improves immediately and pain lessens within 3-5 days, although the full analgesic effect may not be evident for at least 2 weeks. Very low and very high doses have been associated with inadequate analgesia. Common side-effects, including anticholinergic effects such as dry mouth and somnolence, can be minimized by careful dose titration; alternatively, a tricyclic with less anticholinergic activity, such as desipramine or nortriptyline, can be substituted. Alternatives include doxepin and imipramine. If antidepressants fail to relieve the pain of deafferentation, an anticonvulsant drug can be given if not contra-indicated.

Table 7
**Adjuvant drugs**

| Drug category | Drug, dosage | Indications | Comments |
|---|---|---|---|
| Antidepressants | Amitriptyline, 0.2–0.5 mg/kg orally, increasing by 25% every 2–3 days to antidepressant doses (300 mg/day). Alternatives: doxepin, imipramine, nortriptyline. | Neuropathic pain (e.g. vincristine-induced, radiation, plexopathy, tumour invasion); insomnia. | Usually, improved sleep and pain relief within 2–3 days. Anticholinergic side-effects are dose-limiting. Use with caution for children with increased risk for cardiac dysfunction. |
| Anticonvulsants | Carbamazepine, 2 mg/kg orally every 12 hours. Phenytoin, 2.5–5 mg/kg orally every 12 hours. Clonazepam,[a] 0.01 mg/kg orally every 12 hours. | Neuropathic pain, especially shooting or stabbing pain. | Monitor for haematological, hepatic, and allergic reactions. Side-effects: ataxia, gastrointestinal upset, disorientation, somnolence. |
| Neuroleptics | Chlorpromazine, 0.5 mg/kg orally or IV every 6–8 hours. Haloperidol, 0.01–0.1 mg/kg orally or IV every 8 hours. | Nausea, confusion, psychosis, acute agitation. Enhancement of opioid analgesia. | Consider concurrent use of antihistamine (e.g. diphenhydramine) to avoid dystonic reaction to high doses or prolonged course of treatment. |
| Sedatives, hypnotics, anxiolytics | Diazepam, 0.05–0.1 mg/kg orally every 4–6 hours. Lorazepam, 0.02–0.04 mg/kg orally or IV every 4–6 hours. Midazolam, 0.05 mg/kg IV 5 minutes before procedure, or 0.3–0.5 mg/kg orally 30–45 minutes before procedure. | Acute anxiety, muscle spasm. Premedication for painful procedures. | Sedative effect may limit opioid use. Other side-effects include depression and dependence with prolonged use. |

| Drug category | Drug, dosage | Indications | Comments |
|---|---|---|---|
| Antihistamines | Hydroxyzine, 0.5–1 mg/kg every 4–6 hours. Diphenhydramine, 0.5–1 mg/kg every 4–6 hours. | Opioid-induced pruritus, anxiety, nausea. | Sedative side-effects may be helpful. |
| Corticosteroids | Prednisone, prednisolone, and dexamethasone. Dosage depends on clinical situation. | Headache from raised intra-cranial pressure, spinal or nerve compression, widespread metastases. | Side-effects include oedema, dyspeptic symptoms, and occasional gastrointestinal bleeding. |
| Psychostimulants[a, b] | Dexamfetamine, methylphenidate, 0.1 mg/kg orally twice daily, increasing to 0.5 mg/kg if needed. | Opioid-induced somno-lence, potentiation of opioid analgesia. | Side-effects include agitation, sleep disturbance, and anorexia. Giving second dose in early afternoon helps avoid sleep disturbance. |

[a] Not included in WHO's *Model List of Essential Drugs.*
[b] Controlled substance, to be used only by properly trained medical personnel.

Tricyclic antidepressants should be administered with caution to children with increased risk for cardiac dysfunction (e.g. after administration of doxorubicin). An initial electrocardiogram is indicated, which should be repeated as the dose is titrated upwards. Evidence of prolonged corrected Q-T interval or heart block is a contraindication for tricyclic antidepressants or may be evidence of tricyclic toxicity.

## Anticonvulsants

Anticonvulsants, specifically carbamazepine, phenytoin, and clonazepam, may relieve neuropathic pain, especially shooting or stabbing pain. Doses are increased gradually until plasma levels reach the therapeutic range used for seizure control or until side-effects (disorientation, somnolence, ataxia, gastrointestinal upset) become unacceptable. The initial dose of carbamazepine in children is 2 mg/kg orally every 12 hours with an initial maximum 100 mg per dose, which can be increased gradually to 10–20 mg/kg daily (in 2 to 3 divided doses). Side-effects can be minimized by slowly titrating the dose upwards and by monitoring drug levels. The therapeutic plasma level for effective pain relief has not been studied in children. Children should be monitored regularly for haematological, hepatic, or allergic reactions. If the desired therapeutic effect is not obtained with one drug, another may be substituted. However, sufficient time must be allowed for upward titration of the dose for pain relief; steady-state plasma levels are reached in about 1–2 weeks.

Pancytopenia is the major potentially life-threatening side-effect of carbamezepine and may be exacerbated by concurrent chemotherapy. This drug should be used with **extreme caution** in children with compromised bone marrow function and in those receiving myelosuppressive chemotherapy.

Phenytoin is an alternative anticonvulsant; an initial loading dose of 15 mg/kg should be followed by a maintenance dose of 2.5–5 mg/kg orally every 12 hours up to a maximum of 250–300 mg/day. If clonazepam is used, the initial dose is 0.01 mg/kg orally every 12 hours, with gradual escalation by 10–25% every 2–3 days to a maximum of 0.1–0.2 mg/kg per day. Children should be carefully monitored because clonazepam has a marked soporific effect and may cause respiratory depression and behaviour problems.

## Neuroleptics

Neuroleptics – specifically phenothiazines and butyrophenones – are used to relieve nausea and vomiting and to treat psychosis and acute agitation in children. Side-effects include drowsiness, hypotension, blurred vision, dry mouth, tachycardia, and (rarely) urinary retention and constipation. Although uncommon during phenothiazine use in children, extrapyramidal reactions – particularly oculogyric crisis – are feared; the drug should therefore be used with caution. An initial oral dose of chlorpromazine (0.5 mg/kg up to a maximum dose of 25 mg) is recommended every 6–8 hours. The sedative effect of neuroleptics may limit the dose of any concurrent opioid that can be tolerated.

## Antiemetics

Ondansetron is a new antiemetic agent that has proved very useful for chemotherapy-induced nausea and vomiting. Dosing is 0.15 mg/kg IV every 4 hours or by continuous infusion at 0.45 mg/kg per day following an initial bolus of 0.15 mg/kg, with a maximum dose of 32 mg/day.

## Sedatives, hypnotics, and anxiolytics

The benzodiazepines have a number of important indications for children with cancer. Diazepam and lorazepam are recommended for the short-term alleviation of acute anxiety and muscle spasm, while midazolam is often used to premedicate children for painful procedures. However, benzodiazepines cause sedation and may therefore limit the opioid dose that can be given concurrently. The recommended dose of diazepam as an anxiolytic and muscle relaxant is 0.05–0.1 mg/kg orally to a maximum initial dose of 5 mg every 4–6 hours, with gradual escalation as required. Lorazepam is given as needed at 0.02–0.04 mg/kg orally or IV, with a maximum initial dose of 4 mg every 4–6 hours. Side-effects include sedation and depression, and dependence may develop with prolonged use. Diazepam should be used with caution in neonates. The dose of midazolam is 0.05 mg/kg IV 5 minutes before a painful procedure, which can be repeated twice. Although midazolam is available only as a solution for parenteral administration, it can be administered orally if the solution is mixed with flavoured syrup. The oral dose is 0.3–0.5 mg/kg with a maximum initial dose of 15 mg 30–45 minutes before the procedure.

## Antihistamines

Antihistamines are particularly useful for relieving opioid-induced pruritus. Hydroxyzine, which has anxiolytic, antihistaminic, and antiemetic properties, is the antihistamine of choice, particularly for a child experiencing anxiety or nausea. The recommended dose is 0.5 mg/kg orally or slowly IV through a central line, with a maximum initial dose of 50 mg every 4 hours. The most common side-effects are sedation and dry mouth, with occasional agitation. Diphenhydramine is an alternative antihistamine which can be used at the same doses.

## Corticosteroids

Corticosteroids are useful in relieving the pain of inflammation associated with nerve compression, headache caused by raised intracranial pressure, and the pain of bone metastases. Prednisone, prednisolone, and dexamethasone are the most commonly used corticosteroids; dosage depends on the clinical situation. The projected time course for continued steroid use should be carefully considered when it is intended to use a steroid as an adjuvant drug. Side-effects include oedema, dyspeptic symptoms, and occasionally gastrointestinal bleeding. Gastrointestinal side-effects may be increased if corticosteroids are used in conjunction with NSAIDs. Hypertension, proximal myopathy, agitation, hyperglycaemia, psychosis, and opportunistic infections may also develop. Mood changes and weight gain in particular can be profoundly distressing to children and teenagers. After prolonged use of corticosteroids, adrenal suppression may occur and discontinuation of these drugs requires a gradual tapering of dosage.

## Psychostimulants

Dexamfetamine and methylphenidate are occasionally useful to reduce somnolence in children who experience persistent and significant opioid-induced sedation. These psychostimulants may also enhance the analgesic effects of opioid drugs. The starting dose is 0.1 mg/kg twice daily in the morning and at noon, which can be increased gradually by increments of 0.05–0.1 mg/kg to a maximum of 0.5 mg/kg twice daily as necessary. Side-effects include agitation, sleep disturbance, and anorexia. These drugs are usually controlled substances and their use should be restricted to properly trained medical personnel.

In assessing the need for psychostimulants, other causes of sedation must be excluded; persistent drowsiness in patients receiving opioid drugs often has other causes, such as concurrent use of other central nervous system depressant drugs, abnormal metabolic states, or extreme debility.

## Anaesthetic and neurosurgical approaches

There is a limited role for anaesthetic and neurosurgical approaches to pain management in children with cancer. Epidural and intrathecal administration of opioids and local anaesthetics may be useful in children who do not obtain adequate pain relief with oral and parenteral opioids combined with adjuvants, and in those for whom pain relief is adequate but side-effects are intolerable. Indwelling access to the spinal routes eliminates the need for repeated needle punctures, but this is a specialized technique and must be performed by experienced paediatric anaesthesiologists. Deep sedation or general anaesthesia may be used to relieve pain during invasive procedures. In rare situations, prolonged use of anaesthesia may be indicated to manage the pain and distress of the dying child; however, this approach should be considered only after aggressive use of opioids and adjunctive medications and when localized or neurosurgical approaches are not feasible or are unacceptable to the child and the family.

Peripheral and spinal (epidural and intrathecal) blocks are rarely used for children with cancer because of the nature of childhood malig-nancies, which are often widespread, rapidly progressing, or meta-static to the central nervous system. Pain relief from local anaesthetic injections is usually short-lived and repeated injections or continuous infusions are therefore often required. Although they are rarely indicated in children, neurosurgical techniques (cordotomy) in which nerve pathways are destroyed to reduce pain can provide good pain relief when there is localized, tumour-associated pain, refractory to other types of analgesic treatment. In contrast to open cordotomies, the percutaneous approach requires a cooperative child. In highly selected cases, decompressive neurosurgical procedure of the spine may provide relief from severe pain due to cord compression. The choice of surgical or non-surgical management must be based on an assessment of the individual and of the associated risks and benefits.

# Procedure-related pain

For children receiving curative treatment, the pain of diagnostic and therapeutic procedures is often worse than that of the cancer itself. Aggressive approaches to the management of procedure pain are particularly important because children with cancer may require repeated procedures in the future. Procedures performed without adequate pain control can cause anxiety in the child, which can significantly increase the pain of subsequent procedures, alter relationships with health-care providers, and diminish compliance with medical advice.

## General principles

Prophylaxis of procedure pain should involve both pharmacological and non-pharmacological approaches (16). The specific approaches used should be tailored to the individual child, to the specific procedure, and to the needs and preferences of the child and his or her family.

Children must be adequately prepared for all invasive and diagnostic procedures, from finger pricks to bone marrow aspirations and imaging scans. They should know what the procedure is and how it will be done, and they should be prepared for any unusual sights, smells, and sounds. If possible and culturally appropriate, parents should be present during the procedure to provide comfort to their child. They should not be asked to restrain their child for the procedure. Procedures should take place in specially designated treatment rooms and not in the child's room, which should remain as much as possible a refuge from painful events. The competence of the person performing the procedure must be ensured; conscious children with cancer should not be treated by inexperienced individuals who are learning how to perform certain procedures.

Aggressive pharmacological treatment of a child during his or her first experience of a painful procedure is often necessary to prevent the cycle of fear that emerges when that procedure must be performed repeatedly. Behavioural approaches can also be adopted after the initial diagnostic procedures are completed. If pharmacological agents that produce conscious sedation are being used, the child should be carefully observed by an individual whose sole responsibility is to monitor breathing and level of consciousness; pulse oximetry should be used where available. An individual who is skilled at airway management should be present, with resuscitative equipment and appropriate drugs.

# Treatment approaches

Procedures produce pain of varying intensity in different children. In treating the pain, however, it is important to realize that both pain and anxiety may occur and both of these components of distress should be addressed. The approaches to pain management discussed in the following paragraphs are summarized in the box on page 56–57.

## Pharmacological agents

### Local anaesthetics

For procedures that involve needle punctures, local anaesthetics are often of benefit.

- A eutectic mixture of local anaesthetics (2.5% lidocaine and 2.5% prilocaine) provides local anaesthesia through intact skin if applied under an occlusive dressing for a minimum of 1 hour. Maximum application time is 4 hours. This approach can significantly reduce the pain associated with lumbar puncture, venous cannulation, reservoir access, and subcutaneous injections of such agents as L-asparaginase and GCSF (granulocyte colony-stimulating factor). Topical lidocaine preparations may also be adequate.

- *Lidocaine* may be injected subdermally with a small gauge needle or by pressure spray. If a needle is used, a small subcutaneous bleb should be made with subsequent slow advancement of the needle. If lidocaine is buffered with a standard solution of sodium bicarbonate (1 mole/litre = 1 mEq/ml) at a ratio of 9 parts lidocaine to 1 part sodium bicarbonate, the burning associated with local administration is significantly reduced.

## Sedatives and hypnotics

- Sedatives and hypnotics provide anxiolysis and sedation but do not provide analgesia and therefore should not be used alone for painful procedures but in conjunction with an analgesic.

- *Chloral hydrate*, 50–100 mg/kg orally to a maximum of 2 g, is the drug of choice for painless procedures that require the child's cooperation such as scans (computed tomography and magnetic resonance imaging).

- *Pentobarbital*, 1–2 mg/kg as IV boluses to a maximum single dose of 100 mg and carefully titrated to effect, is an appropriate agent to provide sedation in children who have not responded well to chloral hydrate, are older, or are developmentally delayed. It should be administered only by individuals competent in airway management, and in a monitored setting with resuscitation equipment available.

- *Benzodiazepines*, including *diazepam* and *midazolam*, may be used in conjunction with an opioid to provide relief during procedures causing moderate to severe pain (e.g. bone marrow aspirations). These agents should be used in a monitored setting as the risk of respiratory depression is increased when they are given with an opioid. *Flumazenil* can be used to reverse the respiratory depression or sedation associated with benzodiaze-pine overdosage. The recommended initial dose of flumazenil is 0.2 mg as an IV bolus, repeated a maximum of 4 times if there is no response within 1 minute. If there is an initial response with sedation reoccurring after 20 minutes, the dose can then be repeated again.

- *Diazepam* can be used orally at a dose of 0.01–0.5 mg/kg, but it is long-acting and requires continued observation well after the procedure is completed. When given intravenously, it causes burning and local sclerosis but this can be reduced by giving it as a dilute solution slowly through a large vein.

- *Midazolam*, 0.3–0.5 mg/kg orally to a maximum of 15 mg 30–45 minutes before the procedure, or 0.05 mg/kg IV 5 minutes before the procedure and repeated twice if necessary, is the drug of choice for brief painful procedures and is used in conjunction with an opioid. It is short-acting, and the solution can be administered intravenously and titrated to effect, or orally by mixing the solution with flavoured syrup.

## Opioids

For procedures, the intravenous, oral, intranasal, and transmucosal routes of opioid administration are most appropriate. Opioids are often used in conjunction with a benzodiazepine to produce conscious sedation for procedures that are moderately to severely painful. Adequate resuscitative drugs and equipment should be available, as well as monitoring equipment and competent personnel. The two most commonly used drugs in this category are:

- *Morphine*, given at 0.1 mg/kg IV 5–10 minutes before the procedure or 0.3 mg/kg orally 1 hour before the procedure.

- *Fentanyl*, 0.5–2 µg/kg given 5–10 minutes before the procedure.

The combined use of opioids and benzodiazepines should be evaluated for efficacy and for any potential adverse effects at the peak of their action to guide subsequent titration.

## General anaesthetics

Inhalation and intravenous agents that are used to induce general anaesthesia may be appropriate for relief of the severe pain associated with certain procedures. Ketamine, nitrous oxide, and propofol have all been reported as useful in this respect. Subanaesthetic concentrations of ketamine may also be used to provide relief from procedure-related pain, particularly in children with cancer who may require frequent repeated anaesthetics. These agents should generally be used by anaesthesiologists who are highly trained in airway management. Use of local anaesthetics during the procedure can reduce later discomfort and pain.

## Non-pharmacological approaches

Non-pharmacological approaches are an integral and important part of the adequate management of procedure pain, but should not be used as substitutes for adequate pharmacological analgesia in children undergoing severely painful procedures. Cognitive and behavioural approaches with particular relevance to procedure pain include:

- parental involvement

- self-control techniques
- distraction
- visual imagery/hypnosis.

Physical approaches to procedure pain include:

- touch
- cold.

---

**Algorithms for pain management during procedures**

1. **Painless procedures, e.g. computerized tomography, magnetic resonance imaging**

   - Individualized preparation.
   - When sedation is necessary, chloral hydrate 1 hour before procedure.
   - When chloral hydrate is unsuccessful (in an older or developmentally retarded child, or because of an idiosyncratic reaction), and if monitoring facilities are adequate, pentobarbital.

2. **Mildly painful procedures, e.g. finger sticks, intravenous cannulation, venepunctures**

   - Individualized preparation.
   - Parental presence.
   - Grouping of procedures so that repetition — of finger sticks, for example — is not necessary.
   - Local anaesthetics:
     - topical anaesthetics
     - buffered lidocaine.
   - Behavioural techniques, such as bubble-blowing, party blowers, distraction.

---

### 3. Moderately painful procedures, e.g. lumbar puncture

- Individualized preparation.
- Local anaesthetics:
  - topical anaesthetics
  - buffered lidocaine.
- Behavioural techniques, such as distraction, hypnosis.
- Benzodiazepines (in selected children).

### 4. Moderately to severely painful procedures, e.g. bone marrow aspiration, biopsy

- Individualized preparation and parental presence.
- Local anaesthetics:
  - topical anaesthetics
  - buffered lidocaine.
- Any drug regimen that produces conscious sedation in a carefully monitored setting. Examples include the following:
  - *If venous access is established*: intravenous midazolam with fentanyl or morphine 5 minutes before the procedure.
  - *If there is no established venous access*: oral midazolam with morphine *or* oral diazepam with intramuscular ketamine *or* general anaesthesia.

# Spiritual care

Parents need considerable personal strength to adjust to the diagnosis of cancer in their child, to cope with treatments, and to support the child. Individual spiritual beliefs will often provide this inner strength, and spiritual care should be regarded as an important component of cancer care. Spiritual care may prove to be the most consistent and reliable source of comfort for children and their families. Without being intrusive, health-care providers should acquaint themselves with a family's spiritual beliefs as soon as possible after diagnosis. This may provide valuable insight into actions and words that can be appropriately used in the course of a child's treatment, and into particular attitudes that should be respected. Parents and children should be able to choose whom to talk to and share experiences with, rather than having someone imposed on them. True spiritual care must be non-judgemental and respectful, and should help the child and family to find a measure of peace.

# Ethical concerns in pain control

## Care of the dying child

The untimely and tragic death of a child cannot always be prevented, but competent and compassionate care can alleviate a child's pain and suffering (35, 36). Children often know when they are dying, even if this has not been discussed with them; they should receive appropriate supportive and palliative care, including adequate pain control (37). A child's understanding of death varies with developmental age (38). Even toddlers may recognize the word "death", though their understanding is limited and their main fear one of separation; they need reassurance and consistency. Children from 3 to 6 years old can understand that they are very sick and not getting better. Older children can understand that they are dying and are often capable of discussing the fact openly, although they may choose not to or may elect to share their feelings with one particular person. Adolescents are very aware of the implications of the diagnosis, the failure of various treatments, and the finality of death.

Health-care professionals must establish trust through consistent honesty in their discussions with children and parents, particularly in answering all questions about death and dying. Because the disease may be incurable, the child's physical and emotional needs are likely to increase. The child and his or her family should decide where the final days are to be spent – in hospital, at home, or in a hospice. Home or hospice care should follow the same management plan as hospital care, but with parents often assuming primary responsibility for the child's care. Parents need detailed guidance to lessen their worry and allow them to concentrate on enriching and sharing the last moments of their child's life. The publication *Care of the dying child* is a good general reference (39).

Treatment of the disease and associated trauma must include strenuous efforts to relieve pain and must be designed to prevent any unnecessary suffering. This is particularly true in the care of children because they are especially vulnerable; they cannot act as their own advocates, and are therefore dependent upon adults. The two primary ethical principles in clinical care are to do good ("beneficence") and to minimize harm ("nonmaleficence"). In practice, this means seeking a balance between the benefits and the burdens of cancer treatments for the child and family. These principles are founded on respect for the child — the child's right to choose and need to be protected.

The increasingly aggressive nature of cancer treatment involves therapies and procedures with the potential for causing considerable pain and suffering. Health-care professionals and institutions must support the humane and competent treatment of pain and suffering, particularly for the dying child. The health-care professional must also be an advocate for the child. Even when a family believes that the child should endure severe pain, the health-care professional must provide adequate pain relief — if necessary by involving designated legislative or administrative authorities.

## Euthanasia and physician-assisted suicide

Medical euthanasia is the intentional, active intervention by a health-care professional to terminate a life, based on the belief that it is better to end a life of intolerable suffering. The withdrawal of futile treatment, the burden of which outweighs its benefit to the patient, is not euthanasia. Providing adequate analgesia to a child is not the same as intentionally terminating his or her life, even in the unlikely event that adequate doses of pain-relieving drugs shorten life. If the clinical condition of the chid changes, so that treatments once considered to be necessary are deemed futile, withdrawal of these treatments is not euthanasia.

Physician-assisted suicide is providing the means, in this case to the child and family, to end life, with the explicit and mutual understanding that the means will be used for this purpose. However, since it is very unlikely that children will actively seek death if they are receiving appropriate pain relief and palliative care, WHO believes that it is premature to address in this publication the complex issues of euthanasia and physician-assisted suicide for children with cancer.

## Fairness in the use of limited resources

The majority of health-care resources in the world, including those for the relief of pain and suffering, are available to only a minority of children. Even in developed countries, most resources are often directed towards curative therapy rather than palliative care. The aggressive use of expensive chemotherapeutic agents, radiation therapy, or surgery when these can provide neither cure nor palliation represents a misuse of resources. In many countries, a sizeable proportion of the resources available for curative therapies could be utilized to better effect if redirected toward programmes for pain relief and palliative care.

Collaborative efforts already initiated by WHO and various humanitarian organizations should be expanded to promote collaboration between centres in developed and developing countries with the aim of ensuring proper treatment of pain and suffering in children with cancer.

# Professional education

Despite enormous advances in knowledge of cancer pain relief in children, serious challenges remain in clinical practice. There is a wide gap between what is known and what is practised. Health-care workers lack up-to-date information about pain systems, methods of pain assessment, and effective means of relieving cancer pain. The highest priority now and in the immediate future must be the application of existing knowledge on relief of children's cancer pain to clinical practice.

At present, health education curricula (medicine, nursing, psychology) include little information about the sensory systems that mediate pain, the factors that enhance pain, the triggers that activate internal pain-inhibitory systems, or the drug and non-drug therapies that are available for children. The guidelines for cancer pain management provided in this publication should be made available for educational purposes in both developed and developing countries, together with information about the nature, assessment, and treatment of childhood cancer pain. The aims of educational programmes in this area should be to:

- disseminate a common core syllabus containing the essential guidelines for relieving cancer pain in children, with supplementary material provided to meet the needs of individual professional groups;

- provide training programmes for health-care workers in association with their existing professional certification boards and with the faculties of universities, colleges, and training schools.

These aims could be achieved by encouraging and helping societies interested in professional education (e.g. the Special Interest Group for Children of the IASP), national and international medical and nursing associations, cancer societies and foundations to support and advocate educational changes. Such agencies could help to distribute appropriate instructional material on cancer pain management through existing health education systems.

Finally, the public must be reassured that cancer pain in children can be controlled and that there is no need for children to suffer prolonged and severe pain. Drug therapy is the mainstay of pain management but must be combined with cognitive, physical, and behavioural approaches of the kind described in this publication.

# Public education

The lay public can campaign for the comprehensive and humane care to which children with cancer are entitled. To do this, the public needs to be aware that:

- children with cancer often suffer pain
- practical guidelines for alleviating children's pain recommend both drug and non-drug therapies
- opioid drugs are safe and effective for children, when used appropriately for pain control
- appropriate administration of opioid drugs does not lead to abuse and addiction, as popularly supposed
- simple and practical non-drug pain-control methods can be combined with drug therapies to provide effective relief of children's cancer pain.

# Legislative and policy issues

Systems that regulate the distribution and prescription of opioid drugs were established before the value of orally administered opioids in cancer pain management was fully recognized. These systems were developed to prevent strong opioids being misused, not to inhibit their use for pain relief in cancer. The reader is referred to Part 2, *Opioid availability*, of the companion publication *Cancer pain relief*.

Strong commitment is essential to ensure that non-opioid and opioid drugs and anaesthetic agents are available and that legislation governing the professional conduct of health-care workers does not inhibit the adequate treatment of cancer pain in children. A national policy should be established that provides for the phased introduction of a cancer pain relief programme, beginning with the major cancer centres and expanding to include provincial hospitals and community health centres. This will facilitate the development of a structured and coordinated national system for educating health-care workers in the management of pain and other common symptoms of cancer. It should also ensure the availability of the necessary drugs, particularly opioid analgesics, and of continuing supportive and palliative care for all children with cancer.

The step-by-step implementation of such a programme should be continuously monitored and evaluated. Successful implementation should lead to:

- adoption of an official pain-control policy

- consistent methods of pain assessment

- consistent availability and use of appropriate drugs – opioids, non-opioids, and adjuvants

- appropriate use of non-drug therapies

- educational programmes for health-care workers on cancer pain relief and palliative care.

Achievement of these objectives will reflect the degree of success in national implementation of the programme, but the ultimate indicator of success will be the availability and application of pain relief and palliative care for cancer patients in rural community health clinics.

# Organizational aspects

The medical resources available in different countries vary enormously, and the recommendations made here for the organization of cancer pain relief programmes should be modified accordingly. Successful implementation of a programme requires sufficient numbers of health-care workers and adequate supplies of drugs and equipment; it will also depend to a large extent on the willingness of the government to help fulfil these requirements.

The guiding principles for establishing a national policy on cancer pain relief in children are:

- cancer pain in children is a serious problem and one that is inadequately evaluated and treated at present
- children's pain can and should be assessed
- environmental and human factors that contribute to pain can be assessed and modified
- drug therapy, particularly the use of opioids to alleviate severe pain, is the mainstay of treatment
- physical, cognitive, behavioural, and supportive therapies should be used to complement drug therapy
- optimal pain management requires a comprehensive approach to the child with cancer, to control all the factors that intensify pain and suffering.

## Health services

The staff of every hospital and cancer unit should include individuals with expertise in pain management. Responsibility for pain control must be shared by all disciplines involved in patient care – anaesthesiology, oncology, paediatrics, psychology, and nursing – and by personnel concerned with social and pastoral care. Members of the health-care team will advise on, or care for, patients while they are in hospital and should develop appropriate treatment plans for children who return home. A hospital with a cancer unit should ideally be capable of providing all the treatment necessary for control of cancer pain and management of symptoms, including drugs, radiotherapy, and specialized regional nerve blocks.

## Health centres

Although different countries use different terms to describe health centres, all such centres provide essential medical care in the community. They should also provide treatment for pain when children with cancer are treated at home. Hospital care, whether outpatient or inpatient, should be kept to the minimum necessary to establish and maintain an appropriate pain control plan which can then be followed in the community under continuing professional supervision. Health-care workers need to be trained to evaluate children, to advise children's families on the various aspects of care, to understand the principles underlying the use of drugs and non-drug therapies in pain management, and to provide psychosocial support for both children and families.

## Hospices and home care

Palliative care should be recognized as an integral part of cancer care and should make provision for psychosocial support for the family, who are the child's primary care-givers. Additional support is essential for the family and close friends of a dying child. Specialized home-care agencies, hospices, respite care homes, and palliative care units in hospitals exist in a number of developed countries (*40, 41*). Whether they assist a family to care for a child at home or provide a special home for a child, their concern goes beyond the disease and its symptoms to the child's suffering and the factors that affect it.

Home-care programmes to support the family in providing palliative care should be developed throughout the world. Existing palliative care services should be expanded to include specialized services for children, and health-care workers should be trained in palliative care. Government policy should make it plain that palliative care services are an integral part of health care services and should emphasize the importance of developing the best methods of caring for children with cancer.

# Summary of main proposals

## Clinical recommendations

1. Severe pain in children with cancer is an emergency and should be dealt with expeditiously.
2. A multidisciplinary approach that offers comprehensive palliative care should be used.
3. Practical cognitive, behavioural, physical, and supportive therapies should be combined with appropriate drug treatment to relieve pain.
4. Pain and the efficacy of pain relief should be assessed at regular intervals throughout the course of treatment.
5. Where possible, the cause of the pain should be determined and treatment of the underlying cause initiated.
6. Procedure pain should be treated aggressively.
7. The WHO "analgesic ladder" should be used for selecting pain-relief drugs; that is, there should be a step-wise approach to pain management in which the severity of a child's pain determines the type and dose of analgesics.
8. Oral administration of analgesics should be used whenever possible.
9. Misconceptions regarding opioid "addiction" and drug abuse should be corrected. Fear of addiction in patients receiving opioids for pain relief is a problem that must be addressed.
10. The appropriate dose of an opioid is the dose that effectively relieves pain.
11. Adequate analgesic doses should be given "by the clock", i.e. at regular times, not on an "as-required" basis.
12. A sufficient analgesic dose should be given to allow children to sleep throughout the night.
13. Side-effects should be anticipated and treated aggressively, and the effects of treatment should be regularly assessed.

14. When opioids are to be reduced or stopped, doses should be tapered gradually to avoid causing severe pain flare or withdrawal symptoms.

15. Palliative care for children dying of cancer should be part of a comprehensive approach that addresses their physical symptoms, and their psychological, cultural, and spiritual needs. It should be possible to provide such care in children's own homes should they so wish.

## Administrative and educational recommendations

1. National governments should consider instituting cancer pain relief programmes for children, based on these guidelines. The participating agencies should include ministries of health, drug regulation, education, and law enforcement bodies, national associations for professional health-care workers, and cancer organizations. Attempts should be made to raise or reallocate funds for the implementation of cancer pain relief in children.

2. Governments should share their experiences in designing drug regulatory systems to ensure that legislation designed to combat drug abuse does not prevent children with cancer from receiving the drugs necessary for pain relief.

3. National regulatory and administrative practices regarding the distribution of oral opioid analgesics should be reviewed and, if necessary, revised to ensure their availability for cancer patients.

4. Governments should encourage health-care workers to report to the appropriate authorities any instances of oral opioids being unavailable for cancer patients who need them.

5. Guidelines for cancer pain relief and palliative care in children should be evaluated by national cancer centres, with progressive dissemination to the community level.

6. Within the limits of their level of training, health-care workers should be taught to assess cancer pain and to understand its management.

7. Research into the management of cancer pain should be encouraged in ways appropriate to the needs of each country. Such research should include the evaluation of existing ap-

proaches to pain relief and the effects of changes in drug regulation and professional education.

8. Undergraduate and postgraduate teaching, and examination and certification systems for doctors, nurses, and other health-care workers should emphasize knowledge of pain control.

9. Family members should be given training in the home care of children with cancer through the existing community health-care systems.

# References

1. Robison LL. General principles of the epidemiology of childhood cancer. In: Pizzo PA et al., eds. *Principles and practice of pediatric oncology*, 2nd ed. Philadelphia, Lippincott, 1993:3–10.

2. *Cancer statistics review 1973-1987.* Washington, DC, US Department of Health and Human Services (National Institutes of Health Publication No. 90-2789).

3. Magrath I et al. Pediatric oncology in less developed countries. In: Pizzo PA et al., eds. *Principles and practice of pediatric oncology*, 2nd ed. Philadelphia, Lippincott, 1993:1225–1252.

4. Miser AW et al. The prevalence of pain in a pediatric and young adult cancer population. *Pain*, 1987, 29:79–83.

5. International Association for the Study of Pain, Subcommittee on Taxonomy. Pain terms: a list with definitions and notes on usage. *Pain*, 1979, 6:249–252.

6. Melzack R, Wall P. *Textbook of pain*, 3rd ed. London, Churchill Livingstone, 1994.

7. McGrath PA. *Pain in children: nature, assessment and treatment.* New York, Guilford Publications, 1990.

8. Pichard-Leandri E, Gauvain-Piquard A. *La douleur chez l'enfant.* [Pain in children.] Paris, McGraw-Hill, 1989.

9. Schechter NL, Berde C, Yaster M. *Pain in infants, children and adolescents.* Baltimore, MD, Williams & Wilkins, 1992.

10. Ross DM, Ross SA. *Childhood pain: current issues, research, and management.* Baltimore, MD, Urban & Schwarzenberg, 1988.

11. McGrath PJ, Unruh A. *Pain in children and adolescents.* Amsterdam, Elsevier, 1987.

12. Doyle D, Hanks GWC, MacDonald N. Introduction. In: Doyle D et al., eds. *Oxford textbook of palliative medicine.* Oxford, Oxford University Press, 1993:1–8.

13. *Cancer pain relief and palliative care. Report of a WHO Expert Committee.* Geneva, World Health Organization, 1990 (WHO Technical Report Series, No. 804).

14. Stjernswärd J. Palliative medicine – a global perspective. In: Doyle D et al., eds. *Oxford textbook of palliative medicine*, Oxford, Oxford University Press, 1993:803–816.

15. Miser AW, Miser JS. Management of childhood cancer pain. In: Pizzo PA et al., eds. *Principles and practice of pediatric oncology*, 2nd ed. Philadelphia, Lippincott, 1993: 1039–1050.

16. Schechter NL, Altman A, Weisman S. Report of the Consensus Conference on the Management of Pain in Childhood Cancer. *Pediatrics*, 1990, 86(5) (suppl.).

17. Fowler-Kerry S. Adolescent oncology survivors' recollection of pain. *Advances in pain research therapy*, 1990, 15:365–371.

18. Porter F. Pain assessment in children: infants. In: Schechter NL et al., eds. *Pain in infants, children and adolescents*. Baltimore, MD, Williams & Wilkins, 1993:87–96.

19. McGrath PA, de Veber LL. The management of acute pain evoked by medical procedures in children with cancer. *Journal of pain and symptom management*, 1986, 1:145–150.

20. United Nations Children's Fund (UNICEF). *The state of the world's children*. Oxford, Oxford University Press, 1991.

21. Fowler-Kerry S, Lander JR. Management of injection pain in children. *Pain*, 1987, 30:169–175.

22. Kuttner L, Bowman M, Teasdale M. Psychological treatment of distress, pain, and anxiety for young children with cancer. *Journal of developmental and behavioural pediatrics*, 1988, 9:374–381.

23. Hilgard J, LeBaron S. *Hypnotherapy of pain in children with cancer*. Cambridge, MA, MIT Press, 1984.

24. Zeltzer L, LeBaron S. Hypnosis and non-hypnotic techniques for reduction of pain and anxiety during painful procedures in children and adolescents with cancer. *Journal of pediatrics*, 1982, 101:1032–1035.

25. Eland JM. Minimizing injection pain associated with prekindergarten immunizations. *Issues in comprehensive pediatric nursing*, 1982, 5:361–372.

26. Lander J, Fowler-Kerry S. TENS for children's procedural pain. *Pain*, 1991, 52:209–216.

27. Maunuksela EL, Korpela R. Double-blind evaluation of a lignocaine-prilocaine cream (EMLA) in children. *British journal of anaesthesia*, 1986, 58:1242–1245.

28. Shapiro B, Cohen D, Howe C. Use of patient-controlled analgesia for patients with sickle-cell disease. *Journal of pain and symptom management*, 1991, 6:176.

29. Maunuksela EL. Nonsteroidal anti-inflammatory drugs in pediatric pain management. In: Schecter NL et al., eds. *Pain in infants, children and adolescents*. Baltimore, MD, Williams & Wilkins, 1993:135–143.

30. Maunuksela EL, Olkkola K. Pediatric pain management. *International anesthesiology clinics*, 1991, 29:37–55.

31. Yaster M, Deshpande JK. Management of pediatric pain with opioid analgesics. *Journal of pediatrics*, 1988, 13:421–429.

32. Miser AW et al. Continuous subcutaneous infusion of morphine in children with cancer. *American journal of diseases of childhood*, 1983, 137:383–385.

33. Miser AW et al. Prospective study of continuous intravenous and subcutaneous morphine infusions for therapy-related or cancer-related pain in children and young adults with cancer. *Clinical journal of pain*, 1986, 2:101–211.

34. Kaiko RF et al. Central nervous system excitatory effects of meperidine in cancer patients. *Annals of neurology*, 1983, 13:180–185.

35. Koocher GP, Berman SJ. Life threatening and terminal illness in childhood. In: Levine MD et al., eds. *Developmental-behavioural pediatrics*. Philadelphia, WB Saunders, 1983:488–501.

36. Howell DA, Martinson IM. Management of the dying child. In: Pizzo PA et al., eds. *Principles and practice of pediatric oncology*. 2nd ed. Philadelphia, Lippincott, 1993:1115–1124.

37. Stevens MM. Paediatric palliative care – family adjustment and support. In: Doyle D et al., eds. *Oxford textbook of palliative medicine*. Oxford, Oxford University Press, 1993:707–717.

38. Betz CL, Poster EC. Children's concepts of death: implications for pediatric practice. *Nursing clinics of North America*, 1984, 19:341–349.

39. Goldman A. *Care of the dying child*. Oxford, Oxford University Press, 1994.

40. Corr CA, Corr DM. Pediatric hospice care. *Pediatrics*, 1985, 76:774–780.

41. Burne SR, Dominica F, Baum JD. Helen House – a hospice for children: analysis of the first year. *British medical journal*, 1984, 289:1665–1668.

# Recommended further reading

*Acute pain management in infants, children and adolescents: operative and medical procedures. A quick reference guide for clinicians.* Rockville, MD, US Department of Health and Human Services, Public Health Service, 1992 (AHCPR Publication No. 92-0020).

Armstrong-Dailey A, Goltzer SZ. *Hospice care for children.* New York, Oxford University Press, 1993.

Collins JJ, Grier HE, Kinney HC. Control of severe pain in children with terminal malignancy. *Journal of pediatrics*, 1995, 126:653–656.

Finley GA, McGrath PJ, eds. *Measurement of pain in infants and children. Progress in pain research and management, Vol. 10.* Seattle, WA, IASP Press, 1998.

Frager G. Palliative care and terminal care of children. *Children and adolescent psychiatric clinics of North America*, 1997, 6(4):889–909.

*Management of cancer pain. Clinical practice guideline, No. 9.* Rockville, MD, US Department of Health and Human Services, Public Health Service, 1994 (AHCPR Publication No. 94-0592).

McGrath PJ, Finley GA, Turner CJ. *Making cancer less painful: a handbook for parents* (USA edition). Halifax, Nova Scotia, 1992.

Roy D. When children have to die... Pediatric palliative care. A special thematic issue. *Journal of palliative care*, 1996, 12(3):3–59.

Siever BA. Pain management and potentially life-shortening analgesia in the terminally ill child: the ethical implications for pediatric nurses. *Journal of pediatric nursing*, 1994, 9(5):307–312.

Solomon R, Saylor CD. *National Cancer Institute's pediatric pain management: a professional course.* East Lansing, MI, Michigan State University, 1995.

Yaster M et al., eds. *Pediatric pain management and sedation handbook.* St Louis, MO, Mosby, 1997.